THE HEALER'S ART
The Doctor Through History

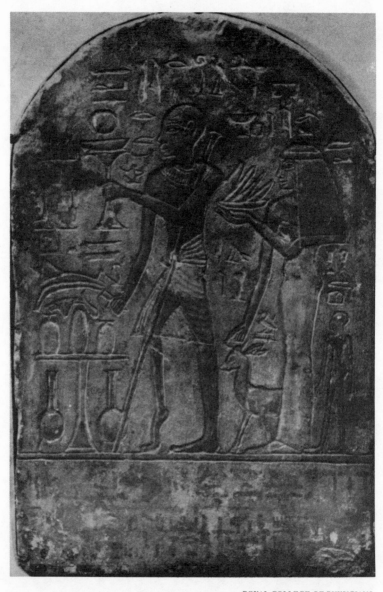

Ancient Egyptian tablet showing an early sufferer from
infantile paralysis

THE HEALER'S ART

THE DOCTOR THROUGH HISTORY

JOHN CAMP

TAPLINGER PUBLISHING COMPANY

NEW YORK

First Edition

Published in the United States in 1977 by
TAPLINGER PUBLISHING CO., INC.
New York, New York

Published simultaneously in the Dominion of Canada by
Burns & MacEachern Limited, Ontario

Library of Congress Cataloging in Publication Data

Camp, John Michael Francis, 1915–
   The healer's art.

   Bibliography: p.
   Includes index.
   1. Medicine—History. 2. Physicians—History.
I. Title.
R131.C235 1977   610'.9   76–54405
ISBN 0–8008–3813–0

Contents

CONTENTS

Introduction

In a way, I suppose, the relationship between patient and doctor has not changed very much during the history of mankind. Today, just as in Stone Age times, it is the relationship between the sick, worried, and bewildered person and the mysterious powers and expertise of the tribal medicine man. The patient hopes the doctor knows what he is doing—the doctor hopes like hell it is going to work.

Though the drugs and techniques available to the modern doctor are more sophisticated than those available in ancient times (though often not as sophisticated as many think), faith continues to play a major part in the healing process. It is important to remember that this faith must exist in the patient and it must equally be present in the mind of the doctor.

This book is an attempt to trace the changing pattern of the doctor/patient relationship through history, from the time when healing was a mixture of magic and witchcraft up to the present day. The journey in between is full of ups and downs, and is a complex weave varying in pattern from doctors being automatically awarded kingship, or even made gods, to being put to death if the patient did not recover. Doctors have been revered, derided, lionized, and occasionally massacred, as happened in the Middle Ages when they failed to conquer the Black Death.

Doctors have constantly disagreed among themselves, and still do, to a degree scarcely appreciated by their patients, who would

7

be highly disturbed to find eminent physicians still arguing about problems which the average layman thinks were solved years ago.

Many doctors in the past have been extremely slow to accept new ideas and have obstinately clung to theories not far removed from the ideas of witch doctors. In America, as recently as 1900, the well-known gynecologist, Dr. Emma Drake, was still advising her pregnant patients to "look at beautiful things and think beautiful thoughts to make sure you have beautiful babies." In England, as late as 1910, the staid pages of the *British Medical Journal* were enlivened by a lengthy correspondence between doctors on why bacon would not cook properly if the cook was having her monthly period! All this makes one wonder how many more antiquated ideas are still being perpetuated by the medical profession.

Paradoxically, the sophistication of modern medicine and drugs seems to be resulting in a backlash among patients and a desire to return to more primitive methods of healing. There is a growing unease regarding modern pharmaceuticals and their almost inevitable side effects and contraindications, the result of which is seen in a move back to such ancient techniques as acupuncture (in America and England), hydrotherapy (in France), and herbalism almost everywhere. Perhaps, as the patient becomes more knowledgeable and less docile, he is no longer strictly patient and becoming more critical. If this is so it is certainly not the first time it has happened in medical history. It happened in 1747, when the noted divine, John Wesley, fulminated against doctors and druggists in his book *Primitive Physick* and urged a return to herbal remedies.

The pendulum swings back and forth. In the following pages we look at some of the extremes to which it has swung in the past, and with this knowledge try and assess the doctor/patient relationship of the future.

JOHN CAMP

THE HEALER'S ART
The Doctor Through History

I

Primitive Medicine

MANKIND HAS ALWAYS suffered from calamities of one kind and another, whether caused by drought, flood, earthquake, or disease. Primitive man, noting the rising and setting of the sun and the moon, the progress of the seasons, the birth, growth, and inevitable death of plants, animals, and humans, did not take long to arrive at the supposition that these phenomena did not occur by chance. To him it seemed logical to suppose that they were ordered by some all-powerful god, or gods, and equally logical was the belief that fortune and misfortune were signs of the gods' pleasure or displeasure.

Gradually there emerged a class of men who claimed that they had special access to these gods, who could interpret their wishes and in this way influence events in their own communities. Fortunately for them, all disasters come to an end and most illnesses abate in time. For the primitive it was not difficult to believe that the improvement in the situation was brought about by the activities of the witch doctor, medicine man, shaman, or whatever other name he came to be known by.

The witch doctor was usually the most intelligent member of the community—and the most feared. In treating illness he noted which plants and herbs of the woodlands were used by animals to cure themselves, and by long experiment came to assess their value on human beings. Certain herbs could reduce fever, for example, and cobwebs could stanch the flow of blood from a wound. The juice of one plant might be used to reduce pain, that of another for inducing sound sleep.

But the witch doctor was also astute enough to realize that he could not maintain his position by the use of medicinal herbs alone, for the knowledge he had acquired was available to all who would take the trouble to seek it out. Side by side with their use, therefore, he instituted a ritual of mumbo jumbo, of dances and incantations, of offerings and sacrifice without which, he insisted, ordinary treatment was useless, for the gods would not be aware of the efforts being made, or would not approve. Only with this ritual could man intercede directly with the gods to be relieved of his sickness or misfortune, and only the medicine man knew how to accomplish this and make the neccessary contact. In time the magical part of the cure became its most important ingredient, and the gyrations, masks, and loud cries of the witch doctor were considered to be the chief means of effecting a cure.

In terms of a time scale we know that medicine men existed thirty thousand years ago. Fossilized remains have been found showing that even as far back as that in time wounds were being sutured by small bone needles, and that boring a hole in the skull was a recognized and comparatively common form of treatment. Today this last technique is known as trephining and is used only when a piece of bone is known to be pressing on part of the brain. That it was common in prehistoric times is probably proof of the belief that a sick person was in the grip of an evil spirit which had lodged in the body, and to make a hole in the skull was the sensible way to let it out.

The association between illness and the displeasure of the gods was a very strong and ancient one. The feeling of awe and wonder at the power of these gods gradually evolved so that the witch doctor became, in fact, a priest as well as a doctor, and the relationship of the priest/physician is one of the most important aspects of early medicine.

Yet though we may now smile at the taboos and complicated rituals used in order to achieve freedom from pain or illness, the part that faith played in the process must not be underestimated. Human imagination and hope are powerful, and to this day much healing is accomplished by willpower and the subconscious instinct to survive. If a man thought he was going to get better because of some ritual, however extraordinary, the chances were that he *would* get better.

Today we know how important this kind of faith can be. More than one religious sect is founded on it, and it can be observed daily in modern medical research in the placebos (inert substances used in place of medicinal substances) used in hospitals during the clinical trials of a new medicament. Here, in blind trials, half the patients are given the new drug and half given a placebo. In many instances not even the doctors or nurses know which patients are receiving the new drug and which the placebo. Yet, in analyzing the results, a remarkable phenomenon is brought to light. Of those receiving the valueless treatment some 14 percent claim a relief of their symptoms as a result. What is even more remarkable is that about 5 percent actually do improve. Temperatures fall, inflammation recedes, and pain is reduced. Though relief is transitory it is enough to demonstrate the strange power of faith, which can cure temporarily if it is strong enough.

It is therefore apparent that the magical cures claimed by the witch doctors are not entirely due to ritual and mumbo jumbo. There are areas of the brain which react to suggestion and affect the body in ways which are not yet fully understood.

Healing of this kind still exists in many primitive tribes today, though the ritual surrounding the treatment has become highly complex. The witch doctor does not only study the action of plants, but also notes which of the tribe's habits and customs are favorable or unfavorable to disease. As an example, in some communities there is a strict taboo against eating cold food. It is possible that this has arisen as a result of observation, when putrefying meat might hold harmful bacteria that would be destroyed by prolonged heating. Another unusual taboo that once existed was against allowing anyone to see one eat, the theory being that harmful influences could be unwittingly introduced into the mouth while it was open, and that the presence of another person increased the chances of this happening. The king or chief of the tribe in particular had to be protected from this kind of contagion, and a case is recorded where the small son of an African chief was put to death immediately because he had innocently come across his father eating a meal. Again, when tribesmen returned from hunting or fighting away from the camp, a whole complicated ritual of purification was embarked upon, lasting several days, to ensure that no malevolent spirits had been brought into the community from outside.

But, of course, there were good spirits abroad as well as bad ones. Each man, in fact, was thought to have a good spirit within him—his soul—which had to be carefully guarded at all times. Eskimos and some North American Indians believe implicitly in the soul, which is supposed to vacate the body during sleep. At times of illness it is thought to be trying to escape, and the resident witch doctor will ensure that the sick person is never left with his mouth open. In the armamentarium of most medicine men can be found a small flask in which the soul can be caught and kept should it manage to leave the body.

In the South Pacific, however, it is believed that the soul is always away from the body during sickness, and that it goes to the burial ground where it consorts with the souls of the long-departed members of the family. On these occasions the witch doctor will assemble as many men as he can, and instruct them to whistle, sing, and play the drums and flute in an attempt to persuade the soul of the sick man to return to his body.

A favorite method of dealing with sickness and disease has always been to attempt to transfer it to some other individual, animal, or even inanimate object. As late as the nineteenth century in America and England, it was customary in some areas to throw some of the patient's urine over the household cat in the hope that the illness would be transferred in this way. One could also wipe the patient over with rags and tie the rags to the branches of a tree to obtain the same result. If a child suffered from croup it was only necessary to trap a toad, prick it so some of the blood fell on the child's chest, and release it, the idea being that the disease would have transferred itself to the animal, who would then go crouping around the fields until his dying day.

Instances of this kind are legion, and remained in vogue almost to modern times. Indeed, it can be said that they have not died yet, as witness the startling claim that copper bracelets can cure arthritis. This, in fact, is a dual superstition, based first on the belief that the copper can transfer to itself the bad influence of illness, and second that metal of any kind is a powerful antidote to illness and misfortune. This is the reason why a horseshoe is considered an emblem of good luck when nailed above the door of a house, and why, in England, sufferers from rheumatism regularly go to bed with a small magnet hidden under the bedclothes. So far there is no justification for the belief, but in 1973 an American doctor working in London was so intrigued by this strange habit of his English patients that he seriously suggested in the pages of the *British Medical Journal* that a series of blind trials be carried out, using mock magnets made of plastic as placebos.

The English may well have some peculiar beliefs, but the oddest theory concerning the transfer of good fortune exists in Greece and Rumania and has to do with the building of new dwellings. It is thought that the soul of a good man can bring peace and prosperity to a newly established household, and that the soul is seen in the shadow. When beginning to build, the foreman therefore looks for a kindly disposed friend, measures the length of his shadow with a steel rule, and then buries the rule in the foundations of the building.

In Rumania the custom becomes slightly more dangerous, as it is also believed that if you give your soul away in this manner you will die. For this reason strangers are often lured past a house which is being built, unless warned off by the cry, "Watch out for your soul!"

That one's shadow is in reality an extension of one's soul is a belief widely held in many cultures, as is the belief that one's reflection is also the soul. This last accounts for the notorious unwillingness of many Asian peoples to be photographed, for the resultant image is also considered to be part of the soul, which has thus been stolen. There is similar thinking in the custom of removing all mirrors from the sickroom, for at that time the soul is well known to be either absent or trying to be absent, and a reflection in the mirror will only make matters worse. It is possible, though, that here psychology rears its hoary head. Most doctors condone this custom and do not discourage it, largely, one feels, because they do not wish the patient to catch sight of himself and be shocked by his appearance. The very fact of being in bed makes most folk feel worse, and few people are seen at their handsomest in such circumstances.

The medicine man, in treating his patients, worked on the assumption that all illness was caused by some outside agency. Not until the time of Hippocrates was it thought that sickness might be due to some malfunction of an internal organ. It was therefore neccessary for the medicine man to ascertain the previous history of the patient—where he had been, what had he eaten, and who had he met—much as the modern doctor does today. The patient may have suffered from a poisoned dart or a snakebite, but equally well his illness could be the result of a quarrel with an ill-wisher who was trying to do him harm by magic at long range. Or again, the patient may have broken some taboo or failed to make an appropriate sacrifice, in which case he would almost certainly be aware of it and would gladly confess it to the witch doctor. This was useful for treatment, as it provided a point of reference, and in any case a confession is often the first step to recovery. The witch doctor, in common with modern physicians, discovered most about his patient's condition from what the patient himself told him.

If the illness was thought to be the result of someone else's malevolent machinations, it was a little harder to deal with, and recourse had to be made to directing countermagic to the other person once he had been identified. But whatever the method adopted, in the final analysis it was only through direct intercession with the gods that a cure could be obtained. If all else failed, then divine intervention was sought by way of an oracle which itself had to be interpreted accurately. Many of these oracles were directed against the accused person supposedly causing the disease, and his chances of escaping were slight. For example, he would be made to drink a cup of a known poison, the theory being that if he were guilty he would die, but if he were innocent he would vomit the poison and come to no harm. This somewhat doubtful method of proving the guilt or innocence of a person (in which the medicine man was not only a priest but also a judge) lingered on in Europe until the seventeenth century, when it was used in the great witch-hunts of the times. The suspected witch would be bound hand and foot and thrown into a river. If she drowned she was innocent, but if she floated she was guilty.

Diagnosis of disease was an important part of the medicine man's duties, but equally important was the cure and the prognosis. In many communities illness was thought to be caused by a spirit entering the body by means of a prick or a "magic shot." The duty of the medicine man was then, with suitable ritual, to suck the spot and draw out the offending spirit which would be seen as a piece of bone or metal. After some time a small object would then be triumphantly spat out, though many witch doctors took the precaution of having a bit of metal or bone in the mouth before they began treatment. The psychological effect of seeing what had actually been causing the illness was immense, and many patients recovered as a result.

As can be seen the role of the primitive medicine man was varied. At first he must question the patient to try and find the original cause of the illness. He must then propitiate the gods by sacrifice or other means before embarking on the cure. If the disease was the result of the actions of a third person, he must be identified and long-range countermagic brought into play. If not, the cure might be accomplished by sucking or some other ritual involving loud noise to drive the spirit away. Finally the soul, if it were deemed to have left the body during illness, must be persuaded to come back.

In certain tribes concern with the soul was considered of far greater importance than treatment by any other means. The witch doctor who specialized in souls was known as a "shaman" and was one who, during his initiation, had experienced some sort of mental illness or something akin to epilepsy. The shaman is a feature of primitive medicine among the North American Indians, Eskimos, and in Siberia, though he occasionally emerges in the folklore of African medicine. His trademark is a drum covered with skin, and he can cure only after he has put himself into a trance or ecstasy, coupled with wild behavior and hallucinations, usually engendered by alcohol or secret drugs.

Because of his violent behavior in this condition, it is customary for most shamans to be tied down before they begin to treat a patient, during which time they often speak in several different voices purporting to be those of long-dead relatives, all giving instructions on how to cure the disease. But the shaman's main concern is getting the soul back into the body, for no treatment can succeed until this feat is accomplished.

Conditions such as these were the backbone of medical treatment for many thousands of years, when primitive man was largely a nomad. During this time he hunted wild beasts for food, believing in a shadowy way in the unseen forces that were shaping his destiny. But gradually, roughly between 10,000 B.C. and 4000 B.C., he evolved from a wanderer into a farmer, living in a permanent place with his family, tending his crops and rearing his livestock.

Conditions affecting his health and hygiene changed with this new mode of living, though the witch doctor continued to wield his influence. Even so, it is only through modern "primitive" societies that we can guess at the real status of medicine in primitive times. We must wait for the development of the first forms of writing, about 3500 B.C., before our theories move largely from guesswork into something approaching factual and accurate information.

II

Egypt and Babylon

IF THE HISTORY of healing is hidden in the mists of remote time, at least the emergence of doctors as individuals can be ascribed reasonably accurately to a definite era. The papyrus reed, used by the ancient Egyptians, together with the development of hieroglyphics, gives us the first true insight of the work of those who were to become the founders of the medical profession. The comparatively detailed knowledge which we have of Egyptian customs and traditions is very largely due to their belief in an afterlife. This belief extended not only to the spirit of the deceased, but also to his body, and it was therefore very necessary that the body should be carefully preserved and supplied with all that it might require in a later existence.

From the period just before the First Dynasty (about 3500 B.C.), preservation of bodies was greatly assisted by the fact that they were buried in tombs in the rainless region of the Nile, where the arid atmosphere ensured their preservation for thousands of years. Buried, too, were scrolls recording events and customs, many of them dealing with medical matters, and these are gradually being revealed as successive generations of Egyptologists carry on their work.

Though our knowledge goes back roughly five thousand years, the oldest manuscripts we possess are not as old as this. The most ancient papyrus found is the Ebers papyrus dating from about 1600 B.C., but incorporating material already known

19

for more than two thousand years. The discoverer of this papyrus was Georg Ebers, a German Egyptologist from Leipzig, who unearthed it in 1875. Fourteen years earlier an American amateur Egyptologist, Edwin Smith, had discovered a bundle of papyri in a bazaar at Luxor. Both manuscripts were of about the same age, and both dealt extensively with medicine, though in different contexts.

At the time of these discoveries detailed knowledge of hieroglyphics and of cuneiform writing had not progressed very far and it was difficult, if not impossible, to ascertain the true importance of these finds. It was not until 1922 that they were finally translated, and 1930 before they were published.

The information obtained threw a dazzling light on Egyptian medical practice. Though it was well-known that the Egyptians were masters of scientific matters and architecture, and involved in complex calculations, it was thought that their medical knowledge lagged far behind these achievements. The revelations of the Ebers and Edwin Smith manuscripts were to prove otherwise.

The Ebers papyrus, generally considered the most important of the two, lists 876 remedies using over 500 different substances as cures. As might be expected, plants feature largely in this, but there are also a number of obnoxious substances, including animal excrement, which were purposely utilized for their nauseating properties. It must be remembered that at this period the profession of medicine was still very largely in the hands of priests, who evolved this method of driving out harmful spirits by exposing them to disgusting substances. The Ebers papyrus, therefore, is largely a mixture of magic and medicine and is less truly scientific than is the Edwin Smith papyrus.

The Smith papyrus is largely devoted to surgical matters and deals mainly with the treatment of wounds. It begins with instructions for healing wounds of the head and neck, and continues down the rest of the body to the feet in an orderly progression which was to be the standard method of dealing with the body for many centuries to come. Yet, though it describes what was done, it never explains how it was done, a fact which makes it less valuable than the Ebers papyrus. It gives no details on how operations were performed and no papyrus has yet been discovered which gives this information. Yet though highly scientific in content, the Edwin Smith papyrus still has its own quota of magic, and one section describes a ritual for "changing an old man into a youth of twenty"! Perhaps this should not be taken too literally, however, and may be nothing more than a reference to the feeling of well-being, and on a par with much of the patent medicine advertising of today.

In both sets of manuscripts religious feeling is high. Various deities are invoked by the doctors, including Thoth, reputedly the source of all human medical skill, and Isis, who provided "magical" cures. Her son, Horus, gave protection against attacks by wild animals. Nevertheless, no god could be invoked without the intervention of the priest/doctor, who thus came to play an increasingly important part in Egyptian medical life.

The very first doctor to be mentioned by name in medical history is Imhotep, who was not only physician to King Zoser, but also a magician, priest, architect, and reputed builder of the first pyramids. He lived about 3000 B.C., and such was his status as a man of great learning that by the time of the New Kingdom (about 1600 B.C.) he had been elevated to the rank of a god, taking his place alongside Thoth and Isis. That the first recorded doctor should have been so honored is significant. Though the status of the medical profession was to undergo many changes throughout the centuries, the idea of a god or king having special powers of healing was to continue until almost modern times and can be clearly seen in the belief in the healing powers of the "royal touch" which persisted in England from the time of Edward the Confessor in 1042, well into the eighteenth century, and was also found in Scandinavian countries.

From the time of Imhotep, medicine in Egypt gradually came to be regulated and codified. Our knowledge of these rules and standards of behavior is gained from the code of the Egyptian King Hammurabi (1728–1686 B.C.), part of which is given herewith:

> If a doctor has treated a nobleman for a severe wound with a bronze lancet and has cured him, or if he has opened with a bronze lancet an abscess in the eye of a nobleman, and has cured him, he shall be paid ten shekels of silver.

If the patient was a freeman the doctor shall accept only five shekels of silver.

If the doctor has treated a nobleman with a bronze lancet for a severe wound and has caused him to die, or if he has opened with a bronze lancet the abscess of the eye of a nobleman, and has caused him to lose his sight, the doctor's hands shall be cut off.

If the doctor has treated the slave of a freeman for a severe wound with a bronze lancet and has caused him to die, he shall render slave for slave.

If he has opened his abscess with a bronze lancet and has caused the loss of his eye, the doctor shall pay money to equal half his fee.

If a doctor cures the broken bones of a nobleman, or cures a sickness of his bowels, the patient shall give the doctor five shekels of silver.

If the patient be a freeman, he shall give three shekels of silver.

If he is a slave, his owner shall give the doctor two shekels of silver.

The rate of pay (or penalty) can be gauged roughly by the fact that the annual rate of pay for a master craftsman was about ten shekels of silver, or two shekels for building a new house. The price of a slave was about twenty shekels, roughly the price of an ass or an ox.

The extracts from the Code of Hammurabi given here are those applying only to the medical profession. The code in its entirety covers practically the entire range of crafts and trades, and sets standards and penalties for each. It is significant, however, that though in over thirty instances the penalty for poor workmanship was death, the status of doctors was such that it was never invoked for them. But mutilation and the loss of hands was bad enough, and presumably kept physicians on their toes. In fact, it is likely that the penalties of the code were never applied strictly to matters concerned with healing, for the penalties were such that few physicians or surgeons would have survived.

The concept of the doctor as part priest and part physician had a double-edged effect on Egyptian medicine. On the one hand medical men were closely associated with nobles and with the court and so enjoyed a very high status. On the other hand their association with religion and the gods created something of a bar to medical progress, as all cures were deemed to be the result of divine intervention acting through the drugs or treatment prescribed by the doctor. Only if the gods were willing could a man be cured, no matter what treatment was given, a school of thought which was to reappear in early Christian times with devastating results for doctors and a violent antagonism against any man-made cures and against those who prescribed them.

A side effect of the Egyptian system was the gradual evolution of doctors into specialists. The original papyri from which all Egyptian medicine stemmed were divided into categories and were thought to have been dictated or inspired by the gods. Herodotus, the Greek historian, tells us a good deal about the practice of medicine in Egypt, and says:

> Each doctor treats only one group of diseases and no more. There are doctors everywhere. There are doctors for the eyes, for the head, for the teeth, for the belly and for other internal diseases. In addition there are some doctors who are not specialists.

The sacred books of Egyptian medicine were derived from the god Thoth, later to be called Hermes by the Greeks. For this reason they are usually referred to as the Hermetic books, though this title is, in fact, an anachronism. The Hermetic books dealt with the following classifications:

The anatomy of the human body
The study of disease in general
Materia medica
Eye diseases
Diseases of women

Since doctors were priests, and since they were usually devoted to different gods, it was natural that they should concern themselves largely with the diseases said to be under the care of their particular deity. From this it was logical that specialists should evolve, and it is significant that in the hot and dusty atmosphere of the desert, the largest section of the sacred writings deals with eye diseases, and ophthalmologists were by far the most numerous of the various medical specialists.

Other specialists had names indicating their particular function, and we find reference to such titles as "the shepherd of the anus" and "the specialist in the flow of inner fluids."

Egyptian civilization lasted three thousand years and more, and it is very likely that during this period both the duties and the status of doctors underwent many changes. Indeed, the strict precepts of the Code of Hammurabi seem to have become modified by the end of the era, for Diodorus Siculus, another Greek writer, in his description of Egyptian medicine just before the coming of Christianity, gives us this information:

> The treatment which was given by the doctors followed the recorded collection of remedies put together by the famous physicians of olden days. If the doctor had observed the rules of the so-called sacred books and had acted in conformity with them, but if, as a result, he did not succeed in saving the patient's life, he was free from blame. But if he acted contrary to the precepts he risked his life.

From this it would seem that if the doctor could not save the patient, even if he had followed the Hermetic precepts, he was not considered at fault and did not have to undergo the penalty laid down by the code.

But doctors did not work alone, though their healing gifts were divinely inspired. Assisting them at all times was a corps of nurses, masseurs, and midwives, the last concerned strictly with childbirth at which doctors were not allowed to participate, though they were allowed to treat gynecological disorders.

Though the prescriptions of the Egyptians were founded on elementary pharmacology, the action of many of the substances used was a very hit-or-miss affair and often several different medicaments were prescribed for the same disease. Compound prescriptions, too, were not uncommon, so creating the basis for the polypharmacy of a later age.

Equally efficacious for the nation's health were the strict rules of cleanliness and hygiene, and in particular the Egyptians' views on overeating (though, unlike the Greeks, they had no formulated ideas on diet). Once more we are indebted to Diodorus Siculus for information. He says:

> To prevent disease they treat their bodies with clysters, fasts, emetics sometimes daily: at times they leave off food for two or

three days. They maintain that the greater part of all the food digested in the body is superfluous, and that diseases procreate themselves from this end, and as these methods which have been mentioned get rid of the cause of the disease, that this is the best means of maintaining health.

Matters such as drainage and the inspection of food and meat were carried out by medical orderlies working under the supervision of the physicians. And last but not least the strict rules governing burial of the dead must have gone a long way to avoid the scourge of later ages which today we term pollution.

Mesopotamian medicine, like that of Egypt, was very largely a mixture of magic and scientific knowledge. The Code of Hammurabi was carefully adhered to, though the methods of diagnosis, prognosis, and treatment differed greatly. Great importance was attached to divination from the entrails of animals, particularly the liver, and in cases of serious illness a sheep would be slaughtered and its entrails brought to the temple for examination by the priests. Though this form of diagnosis could have had no bearing on the disease of the human being involved, in a curious way this furthered the cause of medical research, in that it provided a great deal of information on anatomical structure which was to have such far-reaching effects in the future.

As in Egypt the specialist doctors were defined, but here the subdivisions were concerned more with the method of treatment rather than with the categories of disease. The three grades of medical priests were as follows:

1. The Baru—consulted only to prophesy the outcome of an illness.
2. The Ashipu—used to drive out evil spirits thought to be causing the illness.
3. The Asu—the true physician, or general practitioner, using herbs as a means of treatment.

All three classes were of the highest social rank, working mainly at the court or in the houses of nobles, or sometimes at the various regional headquarters of government. The Baru and the Ashipu were employed by the state as civil servants, and were given a fixed wage. Part of their duty was to give their services free to the poor, but the Asu was at liberty to make a suitable charge. In fact most Babylonians had recourse to all three categories of physician, for rarely was a disease attributable to one cause.

Even the functions of the Baru, Ashipu, and Asu were again subdivided and the Asu, for example, might have to deal with a whole range of malevolent beings varying from the spirits of departed ancestors, through purely spiritual elements to spirits who were the outcome of union between a devil and a human being. All these needed specialist prayer and treatment, and often required the administration of drugs or potions of different kinds.

Doctors in Egypt and Mesopotamia were not paid in money or coinage, for this had not yet evolved as currency, but were paid either in silver or in kind. Then, as now, there was the ever-present problem of the ill person who was too poor to pay the doctor. Though the wealthy and the noble were provided with free diagnosis and prognosis, they still had to pay for medicines and treatment, something which the really poor had no means of doing. Instead they had to go to the community doctors at the temple, or to those employed directly by the state who, as we have seen, had as part of their contract the duty to treat the poor completely free of charge. In this we see, over three thousand years ago, a form of national health service which is still waiting to be introduced in many modern and civilized communities.

Doctors who gave their services free were allowed to recoup their expenses by the sale of drugs and appliances to those who could afford them, and on this they depended very greatly on their dispensers or pharmacists, who were usually extremely knowledgeable on all items of materia medica.

In Mesopotamian medicine the range of drugs was wide, though by no means as extensive as that applying in Egyptian medicine. Nevertheless the drugs and appliances used compare very favorably with modern methods of treatment, and we read of inhalations being used for chest conditions, of sulfur as an ingredient of an ointment for rashes and skin diseases, of laurel water being used for the eyes, as well as bougies, suppositories, and enemas containing many medicinal herbs and plants still found in the modern pharmacopeia.

With their ideas on drugs, on diet, and on a free health service for the poor, the doctors of Egypt and Mesopotamia seem to be much nearer our own time than do the barber-surgeons of the Middle Ages.

III

Ancient Greece

THE EVOLUTION OF medicine in ancient Greece stems from a mixture of knowledge handed down from previous civilizations and cultures. Among these the lore of the Egyptians predominated, and the godlike figure of Imhotep, from whom came all medical knowledge, was transformed by the Greeks into their own god, Aesculapius. Other cultures also contributed to the sum of medical knowledge. The cult of the serpent, for example, as a symbol of healing, came from the Minoan civilization, as did many of the theories regarding hygiene. From ancient Mesopotamia came the belief that evil spirits or devils were the cause of illness, so engendering the opposite belief that only the gods could cure it.

The worship of Aesculapius was widespread among the Greeks, and many of the islands had temples to the god to which physicians and those in ill health made their way. Probably the best known of these temples were at Epidaurus, and on the island of Cos, where their relics can still be seen today. Those who were in control of the temples, the priests and their assistants, were intimately associated with the cult of Aesculapius, but those who were later to be known as the Aesculapiads were, in fact, secular physicians with only the most tenuous connection with temple rites.

The Greek patient, therefore, had the choice of two types of treatment: he could go to the temple for dream treatment or incubation, or he could go to the regular physician. In dream treatment the patient was expected to sleep for one or two nights in the temple, during which time it was likely he would dream. This dream would then be told to the priests, who would interpret it accordingly and suggest a course of treatment based largely on the magic and folklore of the Minoan culture. Treatment by the secular physician, however, was usually based on his observation of symptoms and his diagnosis of the disease, and likely to be more accurate and therefore more beneficial. Dream treatment was accompanied by ritual bathing and cleansing, and the bringing of sacrificial gifts to the priests. Sometimes cures were reported on the spot, but most were considered due to the subsequent interpretation and guidance of the priests. From numerous inscriptions on stone tablets found at Epidaurus, an idea can be obtained of some of the more spectacular cures.

One case on record, for example, is of a woman who was pregnant for five years and who, after sleeping in the temple for a night, was delivered next day of a child. The infant was by then four years old and fully developed, able to walk and to discuss the matter with his mother! The real miracle seems to be how the woman had managed to survive the previous four years, to say nothing of the delivery itself.

Another case of which there are details is of the dumb child who was brought by his father to the temple to be cured. The family was poor, and could make no immediate payment. When the priest asked the father if he would be in a position to pay the fees within twelve months, if the boy were cured, the child astounded all present by saying "Yes" in a loud voice—the first word he had ever spoken.

At the height of their fame the temples of Aesculapius became great centers of healing, health, and hygiene, with baths, entertainments, sports pavilions, and even a theater provided. Even today the cult of temple sleep or incubation persists in Asia Minor and in Cyprus, and religious festivals often include a ritual of sick people sleeping in the church overnight in the hope that they may be cured.

In Greek times, however, the cult of magical temple cures began to lose ground in the face of growing medical knowledge based on diagnosis and prognosis. An increasing number of Greek doctors became available to the ordinary public. The greatest of these was undoubtedly Hippocrates, born on the island of Cos about 460 B.C.

Considering the fundamental effect that Hippocrates had on medical teaching and ethics, it is astonishing how little is known about him. We know where he was born, that he traveled and taught extensively, healing patients by scientific methods rather than by magical cures of the temple. We know, too, that he died at Larissa in Asia Minor about 377 B.C., and legend has it that a swarm of bees settled on his tomb, producing honey which proved to be a specific for thrush in children. (Honey, in fact, has always been used for thrush in children and it is doubtful if its curative properties had anything to do with Hippocrates.)

But the fame of this eminent man rests largely on the writings of his pupils and those who came after him, and close on a hundred books are available recording his teaching and ideas. They are known as the Hippocratic Corpus, or Collection, and embody a code of teaching and practice which seems surprisingly modern. For two thousand years they were available only in their original form and were not translated into "modern" Greek until 1526, when the first full edition of the Collection was published in Venice. The first English translation did not appear until 1849.

Yet, despite this long delay, the teachings of Hippocrates were to have an important effect on medicine and on the doctor/patient relationship, and the ideas of this physician can best be seen in that remarkable document known to posterity as the Hippocratic Oath. One of the many English versions of it is as follows:

The Hippocratic Oath

I swear by Apollo the Physician, by Aesculapius and Hygieia and Panacea, and by all the gods and goddesses, calling them as witnesses, that I will carry out, according to my judgement and ability, the Oath and indenture.

I will honour him who has taught me this art as I would my parents and will make him a partner in my livelihood, and if he should fall into debt I will assist him. I will hold his sons as my brothers, and shall teach them this art if they should wish to learn

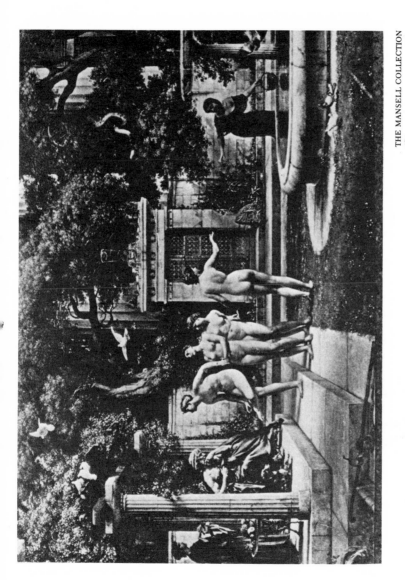

"A Visit to Aesculapius" by Sir Edward Poynter R.A.

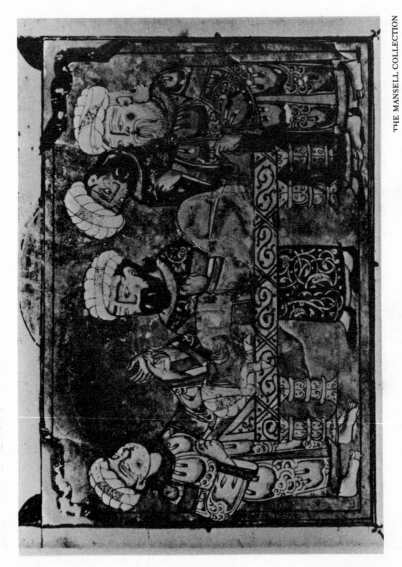

An illustration from an Arab copy of the *Materia Medica* of Dioscorides.
Circa A.D. 1220

it, and I shall do so without fees or indenture. I shall allow my sons and the sons of my teacher to take part in my written and oral instructions and in all other instruction, as well as those pupils indentured to me who have taken the Oath, but to no one else.

I shall use treatment for the healing of the sick according to my ability and judgement, but never to their injury or harm.

Neither will I administer to anyone any medicine which is poisonous, even when asked to do so, nor will I suggest such a course.

Also, I will not give to any woman a means of abortion.

I will ever keep my life and my art undefiled and clean.

I will not cut those who are suffering from the stone, but I will leave them to men who practice such operations.

Into whatsoever house I enter, I shall go to heal the sick, avoiding all intentional wrong-doing and especially every sexual act against the persons of women or men, whether free or slaves.

Whatever I see or hear in the practice of my profession, as well as those things which I may learn in my intercourse with men, if they should be such as should not be imparted to other men, concerning those I shall remain silent, in the conviction that such things should be kept close secrets. Now if I carry out this Oath and break it or not, then may I gain for ever reputation among all men for my life and for my art; and if I break it and forswear myself, may the opposite be my lot.

This oath, obviously intended to be taken by the medical student at the end of his apprenticeship, has been used by the medical profession ever since as a standard of conduct and behavior. Yet it is by no means the only guideline to the doctor/patient relationship found in the Collection. Another Hippocratic writer, in a volume known as *The Precepts*, has this to say:

> I urge you not to be too grasping, but to consider your patient's means. Sometimes give your services for nothing, and if there be an opportunity of serving one who is a stranger and in financial trouble, give full assistance to him. For where there is the love of man, there is also the love of the art.

By no means every man who practiced the art of healing in ancient Greece took the Hippocratic Oath, nor did he of necessity abide by the precepts. Healing was considered a craft, on a par with carpentry or pottery, and could be undertaken by anyone who felt he had a flair for it. The result was that the Greek citizen had a choice of several forms of treatment available to him, from the priests and their magical cures, through the Aesculapiads with their scientific methods, down to the quacks and mountebanks who thronged the marketplace.

Even the genuine doctors, the Aesculapiads themselves, traveled around the countryside, each carrying a staff with the figure of a serpent entwined, to denote their ancient calling. Hippocrates himself is thought to have traveled extensively in Asia Minor and in North Africa.

In most cases the traveling physician was accompanied by a kind of advance man who went ahead to procure accommodation in the village and to announce his impending arrival. Once installed the physician would begin by treating the sick free of charge, partly in accordance with the ethics of the profession, but no doubt partly as an exercise in public relations. Consultation and diagnosis were not the concern of the doctor alone, for the Greek love of argument asserted itself so that both the doctor and spectators, together with the patient himself, entered into a long discussion of the case and symptoms.

Hippocrates gives some guidelines to peripatetic physicians in part of the Collection titled "Airs, Waters and Places" and recommends that the doctor should study the soil and water supply of each village before embarking on any treatment. With this information available, he would have an inkling of the kinds of illness he was likely to meet.

Established physicians, working from permanent premises, were something of a rarity in Greece and were found only in the larger towns. In this situation the house of the doctor was distinguished by the sign of a stone cupping glass, and the doctor attended his patients either at his office or in their own homes. The office was usually in a large house in which lived the physician and his assistants, and there was frequently a private room for a patient or two to stay. Alternatively the patient could remain at home, and in very grave cases an assistant would move in and tend to the patient's needs between the visits of the doctor.

Greek offices were well equipped, with surgical instruments made of bronze preferred, as this was considered to be the most utilitarian and least ostentatious of metals. The instructions for the conduct of a doctor's office in ancient Greece, with their recommendations concerning the best position for the light, cleanliness of towels and bandages, and the provision of palatable drinking water at all times, seem curiously modern. Doctors permanently established in towns were given a government grant for the purchase of premises and equipment, but the traveling physicians depended entirely on their fees and the goodwill of the patients.

Both traveling and established physicians conducted themselves according to the high principles laid down in the Hippocratic Collection. Another very important part of this work was the famous "Aphorisms," in which the Hippocratic code is expressed in the form of a series of pithy and pertinent sayings. Probably the best known of these is "Art is long, but life is short," and a number of them remain apposite to this day. Many of them deal with symptoms, and though medical progress has come a very long way since they were first stated over two thousand years ago, it is apparent that the symptoms of most diseases have remained unchanged during that time, and call for the same kind of relief. For example:

Old men endure fasting most easily, youths very badly, and little children the worst of all.

When sleep puts an end to delirium it is a good sign.

Consumption occurs chiefly between the ages of eighteen and thirty-five.

Bubbles forming in the urine means the kidneys are affected.

In every illness it is a good sign when the patient begins to enjoy his food again.

From the above a good idea can be gained as to how far the doctors of the Hippocratic era had come from the ancient theory that illnesses and disease were due to the displeasure of the gods. Their belief was that illness was entirely due to some malfunction of the body. The main constituents of the body, they thought, were controlled by the four "humors"—blood, phlegm, black bile, and yellow bile, equating with the heart, the brain, the liver, and the spleen. Overproduction of one of these humors created an imbalance and so precipitated sickness. The disorder could only be diagnosed and relieved by close observation and contact between physician and patient.

The importance of Hippocrates and his teaching, therefore, rest on his advancement of three main hypotheses:

1. *All illness is due to some bodily malfunction.*
2. *The environment of the patient must be closely studied to arrive at a satisfactory diagnosis and prognosis.*
3. *Our own natures are the physicians of our illnesses.*

Basically, the last of these is the idea that eventually our own bodies will rid themselves of illness, and that medicine can do little more than supply symptomatic relief—a theory that many doctors subscribe to today.

But not only did Hippocrates define the attitude of the doctor to the patient, he also laid down precepts for the attitude of doctors in all things at all times. He insists that they must be sociable, that they should always look healthy and well-nourished, that they should never argue with other physicians or treat them scornfully. A quick look at the medical press of today will soon reveal how much this advice is now neglected.

The writings of the Hippocratic school also lament the existence of quacks and charlatans, and comment that "In name there are many doctors, but in reality only a few." Among the "many" were some whose role was midway between that of the genuine doctor and the quack. These were the gymnasts, who were engaged in the training of the young in sport and in the maintenance of their general fitness. From observation of the body in action, and from the practice of massage, these men gained an accurate knowledge of human anatomy, particularly of the limbs. They saw the value of exercise in health matters, but occasionally annoyed the established medical profession by propounding that every illness could be cured solely by exercise and diet.

Yet despite the gymnasts, Greek physicians on the whole knew little about the internal structure of the body or how the various organs actually functioned in life. One of the most entertaining ideas subscribed to by the Aesculapiads was that which concerned the "wandering" womb. Greek doctors had a rudimentary knowledge of the womb and its functions, but, as it was apparently the source of new life, ascribed to it an existence in its own right, independent of the rest of the body. Accordingly, to them the womb could move about the body at will, and from its position could affect the neighboring limbs and organs. If the womb moved to the right, for example, the right arm or leg might be affected, and if to the left, the organs on that side of the body. Oddest of all was the theory that if the womb moved upward toward the brain, madness would result. This astonishing theory remained a basic part of medical belief until the seventeenth century, when the anatomists at last began to discover the true function of the organs within the body.

It was a follower of Hippocrates, however, who did most to formulate what we now term biology. Aristotle lived from 384 B.C. to 322 B.C., and was fortunate to work at a time when the dissection of human corpses was no longer banned by the authorities. Though not a physician, and therefore not concerned with the doctor/patient relationship, he is important in medical history as having suggested the basis of evolution in his book *The Ladder of Nature.* He also developed theories concerning heredity which were of value in pointing the way later, and maintained that in human procreation the woman supplied the body of the child and the man the soul. He also took the view that all feeling and emotion came from the heart and not from the brain.

His work was carried on after him by Theophrastus (372–287 B.C.), but the golden age of Greek medicine had ended. After the death of Diocles of Carystus in 295 B.C., one of the last of the Aesculapiads, Greek medicine moved to Alexandria, the new center of learning, where the teachings of Hippocrates were carried on and where they were to exert a profound effect on Roman medicine, at that time in a primitive and undeveloped state.

IV

The Roman Doctor

BEFORE LOOKING AT the varying fortunes of the medical profession during Roman times, a brief consideration must be given to the developments which took place during the short but important Alexandrian era.

With the conquest of Egypt by Alexander the Great and the establishment of the city that bore his name, the cultural center of the Mediterranean shifted from Athens to Egypt. There Greek doctors established themselves and flourished, and two of them in particular made important contributions to the sum of medical knowledge. Both were born about 300 B.C. and both were teachers in the school of medicine of Alexandria.

Herophilus of Chalcedon was probably the first doctor to carry out a postmortem in public. At all events his fame rests on his knowledge of anatomy and his reversal of Aristotle's theory that the heart controlled all human emotions. Herophilus considered the brain to be the organ involved, and also conducted experiments on the nervous system, differentiating between motor and sensory nerves.

His colleague and contemporary, Erasistratus, was a man totally opposed to the concept of mysticism in medicine. He investigated the nervous system even more thoroughly, eventually producing the theory that the nerves were hairlike tubes filled with fluid. He was also the first physician to equate the pulse with the patient's health and considered that the majority of illnesses were caused by an overproduction of blood by the heart. He was violently opposed to the humoral theory, though this concept was not to die out until many centuries had passed. The bloodletting which was such a feature of medical treatment until well into the nineteenth century can be directly traced to the teachings of Erasistratus. It is quite likely that the detailed knowledge of the body and its organs possessed by these two men was acquired as the result of experiments in vivisection carried out on condemned criminals.

Alexander the Great died at the age of thirty-three, only nine years after the founding of his city. From that time onward Egypt was ruled by the Ptolemies, and capitulated finally to Rome with the death of Cleopatra in 30 B.C. All during this time the school of medicine at Alexandria had flourished.

Compared to the Greeks, the Romans were children in their knowledge of medicine and healing methods. Since the founding of Rome in 753 B.C. medical knowledge had progressed no further than primitive superstition. At the time that Hippocrates, in Greece, was evolving his theories and announcing discoveries, the Romans were still making sacrifices and using magic with a complete absence of any scientific thought.

The early Romans had no doctors. Instead, the head of the family treated his relatives and servants by means of simple household remedies and magical incantations, most of which had been acquired from the conquered Etruscans in northern Italy. In times of epidemic or serious illness, the help of the gods was invoked in rituals which, to the Greeks, were utterly bizarre and barbaric.

The first men with any real medical knowledge to appear in Rome were Greek slaves who first came to the capital from the beginning of the third century B.C. These slaves were not doctors in Greece, though compared with their Roman masters their medical knowledge was immense. Noting the condition of medicine in Rome, they were quick to exploit the possibilities of the situation, though in the early days of their arrival the craft of scientific healing remained highly suspect to the Romans. But soon it became apparent that these slaves were having a great deal of success in healing the sick, and their status rose rapidly as a result. It was not long before the possession of a "slave-doctor" became something of a status symbol in Roman households, and the price of a medical slave rose to three times that of an ordinary slave. But it was to be a long time before the art of healing was to be fully recognized, and not until 46 B.C. did Julius Caesar free Greek slave-doctors and confer on them the full rights of Roman citizenship.

In the meantime many of the Greek physicians, already with a high status in their own country, came to Rome to carry on their profession. According to Pliny the Elder the first of these was Archaganthos, who came to Rome from Greece in 219 B.C. and created an immediate sensation by his apparent restoring to life of a man who was on the point of being buried. The Greek doctor was loaded with honors as a result and became famous. Unfortunately for him he was somewhat carried away by his good fortune and attempted a series of major operations most of which failed dismally and caused the death of the patient. There was an immediate reaction against the Greeks and their medicine, and for a period Archaganthos and his medical colleagues were banished from Rome.

This witch-hunt against Greek doctors was led by Cato the Censor (234–149 B.C.), the man who is usually credited with being the first important writer in Latin. He strictly forbade any of his family to have anything to do with the medical profession, and placed his faith in the value of raw cabbage, which, when taken internally and applied externally, he considered a panacea for all ills.

He reviled the teaching of the Greeks in all matters, and said openly that their teaching and medical precepts were having a bad effect on the moral standards of the Romans and were inducing an unhealthy degree of effeminacy. This antipathy encouraged and fostered by Cato, though unable to stop the spread of Greek culture in Rome, retarded it by many years. Pliny himself remarked that "The honour of a Roman does not permit him to make medicine his profession, and the Romans who begin to study it are mercenary deserters to the Greeks."

Eventually the ban was lifted, and Greek physicians once more came to Rome. Foremost among these was Asclepiades, who arrived in the capital in 91 B.C. and charmed all with whom he came in contact with his powers of oratory and persuasion. He was a success from the first, and became an intimate friend of Cicero and Mark Antony.

Though his early training had been in the Hippocratic tradition, Asclepiades did not subscribe to all its tenets. He did not believe, for example, that time or nature were the great healers, but believed in immediate action by doctors in all illnesses. According to him, all treatment should be "speedy, safe and agreeable," and he laid great stress on massage, baths, and correct diet. His best-known theory was that it was the condition of the pores that determined the health of the body, and that if the pores were too open or too closed, illness could result. For him all therapy was geared to affecting the size of the pores by external stimuli. Asclepiades founded an important school of medicine in Rome which continued to flourish long after his death in 60 B.C.

The improved status of medicine which Asclepiades brought about was not without its effect on the slave-doctors. Many of them were given their freedom by grateful masters and even provided with finance to set up in practice on their own. Gradually small societies of physicians developed outside the schools of medicine where, in the Greek tradition, the art of medicine could be argued, and minor colleges and meeting places were built. Eventually these minor "colleges" improved the status to the extent that a few years before the coming of Christianity the teachers themselves were given a small salary from public funds.

The situation of doctors in Rome improved even more during the reign of the Emperor Augustus. He had been cured of a rheumatic condition by his slave-doctor, Antonius Musa, in A.D. 10 as a result of which Antonius was freed from slavery and accorded the rank of a nobleman. In addition, Augustus decreed that from then on all physicians in Rome, of whatever nationality, should be exempt from the payment of taxes.

Medicine had now achieved the status of a free art along with teaching, oratory, and the law, and was not to look back as long as the Roman Empire existed. Even greater privileges were conferred on the doctors by Vespasian (reigned A.D. 69–79), the forward-looking emperor who invented the public urinal (still called *vespasiens* in France today), and in A.D. 117 these privileges were extended yet again by the Emperor Hadrian. These included freedom from any form of public or military service and permission to travel anywhere within the empire at will. Unfortunately many private citizens of Rome felt that this was going a little too far, especially when it was decreed that any family employing a physician should be taxed to provide for his upkeep. The privilege of immunity from taxes was therefore modified so that although a doctor could change his place of residence freely, most privileges were removed if he practiced outside his original district. This effectively stopped what had become a large and dangerous migration from country into town.

In the meantime the medical schools of Rome had been turning out a succession of medical students who eventually took their places in the community. Several forms of medicine were open to them, and appointments under the state were numerous. Almost every public institution had its own physicians, and surgeons were considered of particular importance in the training and care of gladiators. Not only did they have to cure the wounds sustained in combat, but it was the responsibility of the doctor to ensure that every gladiator was in a perfect state of health at all times.

Again, numerous physicians attended court, though only the highest-ranking doctor, known as the *archiater,* was allowed to attend the emperor himself.

At the bottom end of the scale were the physicians who attended the poor and, as a result, remained comparatively poor themselves. Many such doctors gave up their profession entirely to become gladiators or undertakers, both highly lucrative callings, and while the medical profession became overcrowded in its higher echelons, the poor suffered from a scarcity of doctors. Eventually, in A.D. 160, a decree was passed by which those doctors attending the poor were paid by the municipality and were also given preferential treatment if they wished to teach medicine in addition.

Despite the high status achieved by the medical profession in civilian life, there was a curious reluctance to confer the same status on doctors working in the armed forces. Both the army and the navy had a large contingent of medical men, but compared with civilian doctors, their status was a low one. They were barred from attaining the rank of officer, but were classified as slightly superior enlisted men, together with scribes, secretaries, and pay clerks. Even the most experienced and proficient doctor in the Roman army was subservient to the lowest grade of combat officer, and took orders from him. This arrangement is difficult to understand, but probably springs from the age-old mistrust that the services have always had for scientific theory.

The Roman military or naval doctor did not, of course, charge his patients for treatment, though he was allowed to charge them for any drugs or medication used. Though classified as a common soldier he had certain privileges which no doubt compensated for his lowly military status and he was still exempt from all taxation. He also had one important privilege denied to enlisted men in that he could marry while on active service. Without these privileges it is doubtful if many doctors would have been attracted to the army or navy, but in fact many spent a lifetime in the services. Naval doctors were given even greater inducements to enlist and were granted double pay and double rations.

While the Greek influence on Roman medicine was a powerful one, it is to the administrative genius of the Romans that we must look for the development of a state system of medicine and the evolution of their greatest contribution—the general hospital.

The very first Roman hospital had been a primitive enough affair. It was merely an island on the Tiber to which old and ailing slaves were brought and left to avoid the Roman family having to look after them. Any slaves who survived were given their freedom, but many elected to stay on the island and tend their fellow patients. The success of this system became known to the authorities, and gradually small hospitals or clinics were established in Rome, first under private enterprise but later taken over and greatly expanded by the state. At first priority was given to the services and they were mainly military hospitals, being established outside Rome in strategic towns throughout the empire. Near Düsseldorf, for example, a site has been excavated which has yielded an important collection of Roman surgical instruments. Later, hospitals for civilians were established, and civilians were also tended to in the military hospitals during times of peace.

The great period of Greek-Roman medicine reached its climax in the emergence of a man whose teachings were to dominate the art of healing for the next twelve hundred years. This man was Galen, born at Pergamos in Asia Minor in A.D. 131 and who remained an authoritative voice in all medical matters until his death in A.D. 200.

His father, of whom he approved highly, was a brilliant architect, while his mother seems to have been a bit of a shrew. At all events Galen, in describing his formative years, says: 'My father was amiable, just and benevolent, but my mother had a very bad temper. She used to bite her serving-maids and was always shouting at my father." From his father he evidently inherited a high degree of intelligence, but from his mother a dominating personality and an argumentative nature. He entered the school of medicine at Alexandria and after completing the course, traveled for some years in Italy, Greece, and Palestine. At the age of twenty-eight he returned to Pergamos where he became physician to the local school of gladiators. His novel treatment of injuries and wounds, and his unusual ideas on medicine as a whole, soon made him a famous figure and he decided to seek greater fame and even greater fortune in Rome. There he came to the notice of the Emperor Marcus Aurelius, who honored him by commenting that "We have but one physician in Rome—Galen." This did not endear him to the rest of the medical fraternity in the capital city, but Galen was never one to worry about those who envied him. He went back to Pergamos once only, but soon returned to Rome where he remained until his death thirty years later.

However bizarre were Galen's opinions, his views were propounded so dogmatically that there were very few who dared argue with him—and those who did were immediately labeled ignorant by this fiery and tempestuous man. In his day he acquired something of the status that had once been accorded to Hippocrates in earlier times, though there were fundamental differences in their teachings. But there were similarities as well.

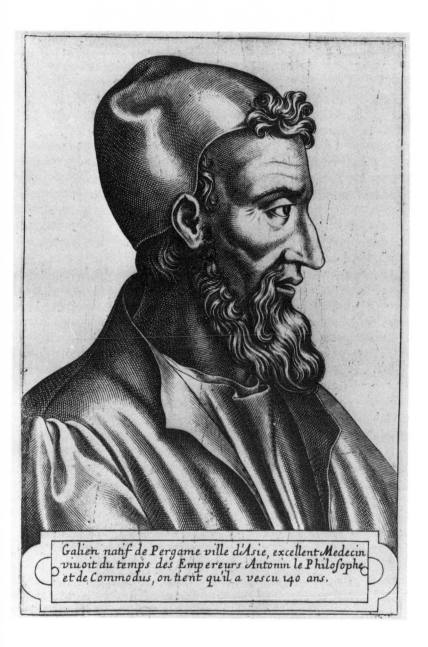

Galien natif de Pergame ville d'Asie, excellent Medecin
viuoit du temps des Empereurs Antonin le Philosophe
et de Commodus, on tient qu'il a vescu 140 ans.

An engraving of Galen

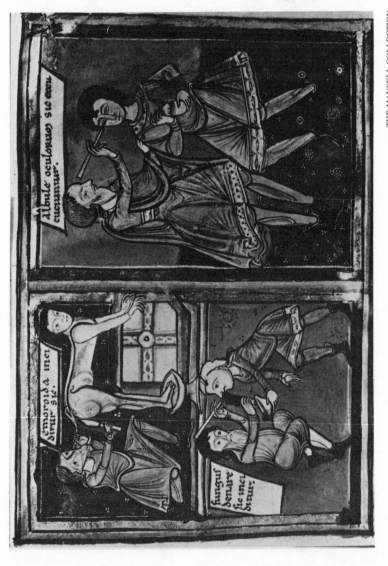

Medical treatment as portrayed in a twelfth-century manuscript.
Top left, treating hemorrhoids. *Bottom left*, removing nasal polyps.
Right, care of eyes.

He believed wholeheartedly in the Hippocratic theory of the four humors and recognized the predisposing and causative factors of many illnesses. His diagnosis was frequently brilliant, as on the occasion when he treated a senator for the loss of feeling in the fingers of one hand. Galen discovered that his patient had recently fallen from a chariot and bruised his neck, and rightly diagnosed that the nerves of the spinal cord had been affected by the blow. He applied a counterirritant to the neck and so cured the condition in the fingers.

But on various other matters Galen was woefully in error. It was unfortunate that in his day the law allowing the dissection of human cadavers had been rescinded and he was therefore forced to study anatomy by dissecting the bodies of animals, mainly rhesus monkeys, Barbary apes, and pigs. The anatomical structure of these animals, though resembling the human body in many respects, was not close enough and caused Galen to assume a similarity in man that was frequently unjustified. Though his analysis of the various sectors of the spinal cord and their function was surprisingly accurate when deduced by this means, his theories about the heart and the circulation of blood were very wide of the mark. While noting that it was the heart that set the blood in motion, he did not realize that it circulated throughout the entire body but stipulated that it ebbed and flowed through the various organs, leaving the heart and returning to it by means of a porous septum. This theory, together with his insistence on the importance of the humoral theory, was accepted by most physicians everywhere and was eventually to retard the progress of medicine by several hundred years.

In addition Galen was a compulsive writer, producing over five hundred books in his lifetime, though less than a hundred have come down to us. Many of these are mainly lists of drugs and chemicals which he found useful in curing illness, and which are still termed "galenicals" to this day.

Galen's views were propounded in his writings with such conviction that they became the bible of medical scholars well into medieval times, and there were certainly none to contradict his teaching during the remaining years of the Roman Empire after his death. In some ways this is surprising, as so often when a dictatorial figure ceases to exert power there are many only too willing to come forward with opposition to his ideas. There were, of course, other writers to emerge, but in the main they confirmed the teachings of Galen. One such was Oribasius (A.D. 325–400), who wrote a digest of medical knowledge in seventy books, and who was private physician to Julian, the last Roman emperor to oppose Christianity.

Another doctor, Alexander of Tralles (A.D. 525–605), who was a Christian, also remains famous for his researches on the treatment of pleurisy as well as for the treatment of internal parasites with male fern extract and pomegranate juice.

But the great days of Rome were over. The empire crumbled and the Dark Ages descended. The contribution of Rome to medicine had been enormous, but it was to vanish under centuries of ignorance as the barbarian hordes swept Europe. When the fitful light of the Middle Ages at last began to illuminate the scene, it was the work and theories of Galen that were first unearthed, with unfortunate results for medicine for many years to come.

V

The East and Arabia

IN THE ORIENT there was no such hiatus. Indian and Chinese medicine have survived, with very little change, from the Vedic Epoch in India (about 1500 B.C.) and from even earlier times in China.

The Vedic Epoch (which lasted until about 800 B.C.) is named after the four Vedas, the ancient Sanskrit texts on which the whole of Indian literature is founded. It is from the writings in the *Yajur-Veda*, or Art of Life, that we obtain our knowledge of medicine at the time.

Its roots lay in the concept of a god or being dominating the fortunes of the family by imposing health or sickness, happiness or sorrow, and in this respect has much in common with most other medicoreligious beliefs. The actions of the gods were interpreted and passed down through priests and holy men, some of whom, as doctors, came to specialize in the art of healing and the alleviation of suffering. The gods of healing in Indian mythology are the Asvins, or Heavenly Twins, who are pictured as riding in a three-wheeled golden chariot and having horses' heads. From this chariot they came to earth to heal the sick, to fertilize barren women, and to prolong life. They were also noted as surgeons, and one tale tells of their replacing the broken arm of a soldier with an iron rod, apparently the first-ever account of a prosthesis.

The Brahmanistic period of Indian culture followed on from the Vedic after about 800 B.C. and was to last almost two thou-

sand years. It is in this period that Greek influences, and later
Arabian, are first seen in the art of medicine. It is in this period,
too, that we meet the first secular doctors in India, doctors who
had nothing in common with the priests and holy men but who
believed (as did Hippocrates) that people are ill because of the
malfunction of one of their bodily parts. For them health was not
a reward for a good life; neither was sickness a penalty for a
bad one. It was not as simple as that.

Brahmanistic medicine is founded on The Books of the
Ancient Three: the second-century medical writer Charaka, the
fifth-century Susruta, and the seventh-century Vagbhata. Between
them they cover the entire gamut of Indian medicine of the time,
with herbs and plants listed by the hundred as well as a formidable list of animal and mineral remedies.

The Book of Susutra is very strong on surgery, and surprisingly comprehensive in view of the fact that the religious laws
of the time banned the dissection of human bodies. Intestinal
operations were performed, however, and sutures made in an
ingenious process by which giant black ants were used to bite
the edges of the wound together, after which their bodies were
cut off, leaving the head to form a permanent "stitch." The only
circumstances under which a dead body could be cut was the
removal of a child from its dead mother by means of Caesarean
section. Unlike the situation existing in many other cultures and
later Christian communities, the surgeon always enjoyed superior
status and was inevitably a member of a high caste.

The training of medical students in Brahmanistic times was
rigorous and strictly controlled. The center and focus of all
medical knowledge was the holy city of Benares, as, indeed, it
was the focal center of all Indian learning. Students could apply
to become the pupils of selected medical men, but it did not
always follow that they would be accepted. Preference was given
to the sons of physicians and great attention paid to the appli-
cant's morals, his state of health, and his spiritual qualities.
Training was for six years, from the twelfth to the eighteenth
year of age, and at the acceptance ceremony the candidate had
to promise to obey the teacher in all things, to grow a beard, and
not to eat meat.

By the end of the sixth year the budding physician had learned all his master could teach him and was ready for the final ceremony. In this he had to promise to utilize his medical knowledge in accordance with a complicated medical code outlined by the local rajah, who, in the event, was the one who decided whether or not the candidate had satisfied the examiners. He was not allowed to give medical treatment to hunters, criminals, or incurables, or to those who had lost caste. No fees should be demanded of priests, relatives, or the poor, and doctors were exempt from all taxes due on the proceeds of their profession.

From the wealthy, fees should be extracted in accordance with their standing, and should a patient refuse to pay a doctor after a certain length of time, his entire possessions went to the physician by law. There was, therefore, every inducement to pay promptly. It can therefore be seen that in India the medical profession at the time had a higher status than was found in virtually any other country.

Owing to the belief in the transmigration of souls from human to animal, there was no differentiation between human and veterinary medicine. The height of ambition for a young doctor was to be appointed as a court physician and look after the health of the rajah and his holy cows. Though one odd result of belief in a continuing life was that an illness suffered in this life could be a punishment for some sin committed in a previous existence.

The organization of health and the theory of sickness were very different in ancient China. Here the basic philosophy of health was embodied in the principles of Yin (female) and Yang (male) described by the Emperor Fu Hsi in 2900 B.C. There was no question here of any gods punishing the evildoer by sickness for his transgressions. The Yin principle was feminine, dark, passive, and cold, while Yang was male, bright, positive, and warm. Every living thing was composed of these two principles harmoniously balanced, and in this way the universe was controlled. Any illness was due to these two factions being temporarily out of balance, a proposition formulated by the real founder of Chinese medicine, the "Yellow Emperor" Huang-Ti (2600 B.C) in his monumental book called *The Theory of Internal Diseases.*

In the early years of Chinese culture the status of medicine was at its highest, and it is from this period that come the basic diagnostic and therapeutic techniques of pulse-taking and acupuncture. Many high-born princes interested themselves in medicine, including Chang Chung-Ching (about A.D. 200), sometimes called the Hippocrates of Chinese medicine, and Huan-T'uo (A.D. 190–268), one of the few Chinese surgeons.

The art of diagnosis by pulse-taking was taught in all Chinese medical schools, and the course was long and difficult. Fifty-one different kinds of pulse beat were identifiable, taken at eleven different points on the body and each pointing to a separate medical condition. That this technique had much to commend it is proved by a recent test when a party of French doctors in China diagnosed the illnesses of hospitalized patients by conventional Western means, and Chinese doctors (who had not previously attended the patients) attempted diagnosis purely by reference to the pulse. Their findings coincided in 80 percent of the cases.

Diagnosis was also carried out by examination of the color of the tongue, and it was said that there were thirty-seven possible shades to indicate the condition of the patient and the probable duration of the disease.

As for treatment, it is the ancient technique of acupuncture (at least five thousand years old) that has recently captured the imagination of Western doctors and caused them to study the system more closely. According to the Yellow Emperor's classic book on internal medicine, acupuncture points are distributed symmetrically about the body. The number of points varies, according to which authority you read, but the Hungarian writer Stephan Palos, in his *The Chinese Art of Healing* (1971), says some 722 points are today generally acknowledged. Widely separated points affect the working of the same organ. All points affecting the same organ are interconnected by lines called meridians. There are said to be twenty-four meridians as well as some others which affect not the internal organs but the skin and muscle.

According to Palos: "All these meridians have a definite functional character, depending on whether they affect organs, muscle or skin. Knowledge of the interconnection between the surface of the skin and the internal organs is the unique and special discovery of Chinese Medicine." The theory behind acupuncture is that energy passes along the meridians, thus correcting the balance of the organ (the Yin and Yang). The energy is activated at the point of puncture by special needles of varying kinds.

In ancient times nine varieties of needle were used, though strictly speaking not all were needles, for some had a triple cutting edge and some were miniature lances. Today most needles are made of gold, silver, or steel alloy, though many Western practitioners say that the metal itself is unimportant. In 1957, however, a Rumanian doctor claimed to have proved differing physiological activity (including increased production of bile) according to the metal used, and claimed gold to be the most valuable.

Needles are inserted to a depth of three to ten millimeters, though in China many patients make use of a kind of do-it-yourself technique for minor ailments which consists of pressing strongly with one finger on the appropriate acupuncture point, the most important of which they know.

According to Palos the first general summary of results achieved by acupuncture was made in China in 1954, during which eight thousand cases were evaluated. The success rate was given as 92.5 percent.

Closely associated with acupuncture is treatment by the moxa method, usually termed moxibustion. In this technique heat is applied to the point, and it is possible that this method predates the use of needles and was already in use in the Stone Age. Certainly the healing effect of heat has been used from the most ancient times, and the Yellow Emperor refers to it as a highly developed mode of treatment. In its most common form the leaves of the mugwort (or moxa) plant are burned in a small container immediately above the appropriate acupuncture point, though certain points are reserved only for acupuncture and others only for moxibustion. Garlic and ginger are sometimes used as alternatives to mugwort.

Because of the great fear of blood displayed by the Chinese, surgery remained at a low ebb in ancient times, as did dentistry. The dissection of human cadavers was banned and obstetrics remained firmly in the hands of midwives. In other respects Chinese medicine was well in advance of its Western counterpart, and already, in the eleventh century, preventive inoculation against smallpox was being used. It was to be another seven hundred years before this method was introduced to Europe via Turkey by Lady Mary Wortley Montagu, and engaged the attention of Edward Jenner.

By the fourteenth century medicine was highly organized in China, and thirteen separate branches of the healing art had become established. Wealthy families had their own private physicians who were paid as long as the family was well, but made to work for nothing during periods of illness, thus providing a powerful incentive to keep the family free from disease.

During the period of the Yüan emperors (1280–1368) women were allowed to become medical students for the first time. By the time of the Manchu Dynasty (1644–1912), Chinese medicine had ceased to move forward, and interest was being expressed in the medicine of the West which had been introduced by the Jesuit missionary, Johann Schreck, who had come to China from Switzerland in 1621. But the Chinese authorities, as a whole, were not in favor of any ideas from Europe and it was not until 1828, when American and British missionaries at last succeeded in penetrating to the interior, that conditions for modern medicine improved appreciably.

After the founding of the Chinese Republic by Sun Yat-sen in 1912, Chinese and European medicine really became integrated and the modern Chinese Medical Association was formed. But the training of doctors proceeded very slowly, as few could be attracted to the profession, and even by 1948 there was still only one doctor in China to twenty thousand patients.

Though modern medical methods were introduced, the Chinese continued to display great faith in their ancient herbal heritage. This is still so today, where modern drugs are manufactured and advertised to doctors side by side with the herbal remedies of centuries ago. This juxtaposition of old and modern medicine applies equally to Japan, where the first Chinese doctors appeared in the third century. During the years that followed, most Japanese medical students were sent to China to study, where the course lasted a minimum of seven years. In 1549 a Spanish Jesuit missionary, Francis Xavier, landed in Japan and began to instill the rudiments of European medicine into the community, though his stay lasted only two years. No further progress was made until 1771, when the Dutch East India Company established a base in Nagasaki. Here, for the first time, Japanese doctors were present at the dissection of a human body and were able to see that it was exactly as described in European medical textbooks, and not as in their own books. From that moment every European medical book available was translated into Japanese, and the medical link with China was largely severed. The final emergence of Japanese medicine came in 1902, with the alliance with Great Britain and the incorporation of the Japanese Medical Academy into the University of Tokyo.

While medicine in the Far East was evolving, Islamic and Arabian medicine was exerting its influence on the Europe of the Middle Ages. It is to the Moslem Empire that we must look to discover the reason why Greek medicine was not wholly lost, for the Arabs very early on began translating the Greek medical writers, and so preserving their thoughts and precepts, during a period when cultural darkness was settling over Europe. Curiously enough the work was initiated by a Christian doctor, Nestorius, banished from Constantinople for heresy in A.D. 431. For two centuries his followers, the Nestorians, continued their highly important task of translating into Arabic every Greek medical manuscript they could obtain. It should be remembered, though, that in this context the word Arabian refers only to the language used, for the Moslem Empire, eventually extending from Samarkand to Spain, embraced many forms of religion and many ethnic cultures. Comparatively few of the many Arab writers were, in fact, pure Arabians.

One of the great contributions made by the Arabs to medicine was in materia medica, or pharmacology, and several new drugs were discovered by them whose names remain in the pharmacopéia today. The word drug itself is of Arabic origin, as are such words as alcohol, alkali, and sugar. They also investigated fevers, and in particular diseases of the eye, endemic in the Near East. They were also greatly concerned with chemistry, or alchemy, and expended much time and energy in seeking to transmute base metal to gold and in the search for the elixir of life. A well-known Arabian physician of the times was the Syrian, Gabriel Baktishua, one of a dynasty of doctors and personal physician to Harum-al-Rashid (764–809), the most famous of the caliphs of Baghdad. Baktishua was probably one of the wealthiest doctors of all time, and is said to have received on one occasion the equivalent, in modern coinage, of fifty thousand dollars for affecting a single cure. Small wonder that when he died he is estimated to have left the equivalent of ten million dollars.

The first Arabian doctor to achieve worldwide fame, however, was abu-Bakr Muhummad ibn-Zakariya al-Razi (850–923), whose modern name is thankfully rendered as Rhazes. He was born in Teheran and began life as a musician, embracing medicine when he was past forty years of age. After qualifying as a doctor he moved to Baghdad, where one of his first tasks was to decide the location of a new hospital. Rhazes hung pieces of meat at various points in the city, and eventually sited the hospital at the point where the putrefaction of the meat was longest delayed. During his life he wrote about 140 medical textbooks and was the first doctor to differentiate between smallpox and measles. His works include such useful sections as "Medical Hints for Travelers" and "Advice on Buying Slaves." When, in old age, his eyesight began to fail, he refused to undergo an operation on the grounds that he had already seen too much suffering during his life.

The man who was later to be named the Arabian Prince of Physicians was abu-ali al-Husayn ibn-Sina, whose modern name is Avicenna (980–1037). He was something of an infant prodigy, and by the age of ten was said to be capable of reciting the whole of the Koran by heart. From this auspicious beginning he grew up to be a somewhat flamboyant character and was appointed court physician at Baghdad at the age of seventeen.

He wrote prodigiously and traveled extensively, and became noted as a lover of wine and women as well as for his undoubted medical knowledge and skill.

His five-volume *Canon of Medicine* is still used extensively in the Middle East today and contains many pertinent aphorisms which are still valid. Among these are: "Extreme pain in the abdomen, with fever, is serious" and "If a patient makes movements with his hands as if picking things off himself, it is a sure sign of death."

He also gave instruction and much general information on health and hygiene, the best means of selecting a site for a house, the effect of climate on health, and hints for looking after aged relatives. There is also a surprisingly up-to-date section on the therapeutic use of music in the sickroom.

Avicenna's life was comparatively short, if merry, and there is evidence that alcoholism hastened his end. His forthright writings put him on a par with Galen, and his influence was such that his books remained standard reading for students until well into the seventeenth century.

In Spain, the western limit of the Islamic Empire and known as the Western Caliphate, Arabian medicine also exerted a great deal of influence. In this area one doctor who achieved fame far outside the boundary of his native land was Avenzoar (1091–1162), who was born in Seville. He was a leader in the movement against quackery and superstition in medicine, rife at the time, and is credited with having discovered the existence of the mite causing scabies. He wrote at least six important medical textbooks, of which three survive, one of which includes the advice that for healing a rupture the only treatment is two months' bedrest, together with a diet of baked bread and boiled sparrows.

Another doctor/philosopher in Spain was Rabbi Moses ben Maimon (1135–1204), usually known as Maimonides. He spent much time in Egypt, where he was court physician to Saladin, the sultan, the archenemy of the Anglo-French King Richard Coeur de Lion, and is thought to be the original El Hakim, featured in Sir Walter Scott's novel, *The Talisman*. Maimonides wrote many books on hygiene, on the formation of character by clean living, and on the treatment of poisons. His many teachings were based on the importance of the dual care of the soul as well as of the body. His famous *Guide for the Perplexed* is an essay on how medicine can be reconciled with religion and is the only one of his books available in an English translation.

The Arabian Empire produced many great teachers and medical thinkers, and was also famous for the standard of its hospitals, the most important of which were at Cordova (Spain), Damascus, and Cairo. But by the beginning of the thirteenth century the great days of the empire were coming to an end. Cordova was sacked by the Moors in 1236, Baghdad by the Mongols in 1258, yet the learning and erudition of Islam were not to be lost. They gravitated to the university city of Salerno, near Naples, which had been the first medical school in Europe, and took root. There they flowered again, in an ambience which made Salerno the natural meeting place of active minds of every nationality, and was to come to full bloom in the period of the Renaissance, two centuries later.

VI

From the Romans to the Middle Ages

COMPARED WITH the knowledge we have of Egyptian, Greek, and Roman medicine, information on medical matters at the dawn of Christianity is sparse. What is observable from the study of the writings of the times is that the status of the physician underwent a sad decline during this period. The early Christian Church had no great liking for doctors, and indeed at times was expressly hostile to them.

This hostility was based on two main precepts. First was the idea that illness and misfortune somehow purified the soul and prepared it for the joys of the hereafter. Second, that all illnesses were sent by God, and it was therefore impudent, if not downright blasphemous, to try and cure them by purely natural means.

Yet even before the coming of Christ there had been some rumblings against the medical profession, and as far back as 180 B.C. a noted Jewish writer, Jesus, son of Sirach, introduced a note of skepticism in his famous *In Praise of Physicians* when he said: "A long illness baffles physicians; the king of today will be dead tomorrow." Job's opinion of doctors (though in fairness to him he may well have been biased) is well-known and is often quoted: "You are forgers of lies; you are physicians of no value" (Job 13:4).

Though we have no Jewish equivalent of the Ebers and Edwin Smith papyri, Old Testament writings give us certain clues to the status of doctors in Biblical times. A good deal of

Jewish medical knowledge and customs can be traced directly back to the Egyptians, in particular their ideas on sanitation and hygiene. But Jewish doctors had a different kind of status which was very much lower than that of their Egyptian counterparts. One fact which influenced them was that in Jewish society the doctor, for the first time, was not considered a priest. He existed and earned his living solely as a medical practitioner, though still having recourse to a certain amount of magic in his diagnoses and prescriptions, even if not directly connected with religious matters. In fact temple doctors still existed, though in a very different sense from before. These were now doctors who went to the temple to treat the priests themselves, who suffered from the occupational disorder of stomach cramps and colds due to excessive washing, scanty clothing, and walking on the cold flagstones in bare feet.

We also know that Jewish physicians were paid, for we read in Exodus, "if men strive together, and one smite another with a stone, or with his fist, and he die not but keepeth to his bed: if he rise again and walk abroad upon his staff, then shall he that smote him be quit: only shall he pay for the loss of time and the physician's fee."

In later years there was still a certain amount of mistrust for doctors among the Jews. A writer warns: "Do not dwell in a town whose chief citizen is a physician," adding darkly: "Drink no medicine. . . . Stir up no snakes."

Those who later recorded the ministry of Jesus Christ also found plenty of antidoctor ammunition. Christ's miraculous cures performed merely by the laying on of hands were taken as proof that all illness and disease came from God and could be cured only by Him. Not until the emergence of that curious medieval mystic, Hildegard of Bingen (1098–1179) did a religious teacher advocate temporal methods of healing, with the ingenious argument that all means should be adopted to keep the body healthy and free from disease, as a sick body was more easily ensnared by Satan and his minions.

Yet many doctors in the early Christian era were accepted, even by Christians, and the author of the Acts of the Apostles himself, Luke, was said to be a painter and a physician. For this reason many modern religious societies bear the name "St. Luke," though some prefer one of the names of the brothers, Cosmas and Damian, early Christians who were butchered as much for their calling as doctors as for their faith, and who gave their names to the first recorded professional medical association to be formed in 1567.

Cosmas and Damian were martyred about A.D. 300. Two hundred years later Emperor Justinian venerated them and established a special church of healing for their worship at Constantinople. Here was practiced the ancient form of healing already old at the time of Aesculapius—"church sleep" or healing by dreams. The patient went to the church for several successive nights to sleep, during which it was hoped he would have a dream in which Cosmas and Damian would appear to him and give him instructions for healing his condition and which he could pass on to the doctors. Sometimes the faith of the patient was such that a "miracle" was reported. Church sleep was considered particularly beneficial in cases of swollen glands and stomach ulcers, both conditions amenable to what we today term psychosomatic treatment. The medical brothers became, in time, not only the patron saints of physicians and surgeons, but also of wet nurses, midwives, apothecaries, and, for some unknown reason, haberdashers.

The most interesting legend concerning Cosmas and Damian is of the man who had a gangrenous leg and who went for a period of church sleep in Rome. The saintly brothers came to him in a dream and told him to seek a surgeon and instruct him to amputate the leg just below the knee. The surgeon was then to amputate the good leg of another patient who was dying and put it in its place. The man sought out a surgeon and told him of his dream, and the amputations and transplant were carried out accordingly. Unfortunately the dying donor of the healthy leg was a black man, the result being that the gangrenous patient ended up with two good legs, one white and one black.

The general mistrust of ordinary physicians during the Dark Ages and the Christian insistence that illness could be cured only by divine intervention resulted in medicine being confined mainly to the monasteries and convents. The effect was to cause the sick to be gathered together in religious communities, an arrangement which was the foundation of the modern hospital system. The first hospital was constructed by Basil, bishop of Caesarea, about A.D. 370, which included not only beds for the sick, but also accommodation for the poor, homes for the aged, and a special section for the inevitable lepers. Unfortunately, as had happened in Egypt, too close a relationship between medicine and religion had the effect of stifling medical progress, and the discoveries and teachings of the Greeks were largely wasted.

Yet it is paradoxical that the so-called Dark Ages were directly responsible for three great medical institutions—the establishment of hospitals, the creation of universities with medical schools, and the beginnings of concern with public health. Though the age was dark, medicine was brought gradually into the light, and Theodoric the Great, king of the Ostrogoths (a term still used to indicate a barbarian in France), took over the remnants of Roman medicine in about A.D. 500, revised their medical laws and maintained a high standard of professionalism for doctors generally. In these non-Christian communities religious considerations did not arise, and in their treatment of the sick, the poor, and the aged, they showed far more charity and compassion than did their Christian contemporaries.

As Christianity gradually penetrated throughout Europe, it was affected by these enlightened attitudes, and Aurelius Cassiodus (490–583), the Roman convert who succeeded Theodoric as chancellor of the Goths and later became a Benedictine monk, established a place of learning in southern Italy where the language of the Greeks still survived. Here he set his monks translating medical treaties from the original Greek into Latin to be used for the training of physicians and surgeons.

The Visigoths, who flourished in the south of France until A.D. 507 and in Spain until A.D. 711, also had high medical standards, and their laws governing the treatment of disease and the activities of doctors were almost as severe as that of the Hammurabi Code, though they did not recommend death or mutilation. The pay of the physician was not stipulated, but this had to be arranged with the family of the patient before treatment could start, and the physician was expected to provide a security. If the patient died all fees were canceled, though the family kept the security. Surgeons, however, did have a definite scale of fees, including, for example, the sum of ten dollars for an operation for cataract of the eye. Bloodletting was a favorite method of treatment (and was to remain so until well into the nineteenth century), but if the patient suffered any ill effects from this, the doctor had to pay the very large fine of about two hundred dollars. If the patient died as a result of these activities, no fine was imposed, but the wretched surgeon was delivered into the hands of the sorrowing relatives for suitable treatment! If it was a slave or serf who died, then the surgeon had to compensate his master.

The Visigoth code regarding medical treatment of women was strict, for the Visigoths themselves were very conscious of the sexual excesses which had been committed by their own people in the past. No freewoman could be treated by a doctor alone, but only in the presence of neighbors or relatives, in order that the doctor should have no opportunity for "immoral jests." If he offended in this respect he was liable to a fine of twenty-five dollars (a comparatively small sum which some doctors may have thought to be worth the risk). There were also rules governing the treatment of the sick who were in prison, and no doctor could treat such a patient without a warder attending in case the doctor supplied a poison by which the prisoner could cheat the gallows or executioner. Doctors themselves were never thrown into prison unless it was a clear case of murder, though for all other offenses they stood their trial and paid the penalty exactly as other members of the community.

From this it can be seen that, though attempts were made to raise the standards of medical behavior, doctors were still deeply mistrusted, so not many capable men were attacted to the profession, which left the field open to a growing number of charlatans and quacks.

The death penalty for medical neglect was reimposed by the Merovingians (481–751), and body surgeons and those serving the court must have gone in fear of their lives. As an example, in the year 580, Queen Austrichildia, wife of the Frankish King Guntram, was suffering from dysentery and was being attended to by two doctors. Fearing that not enough effort was being made to save her, she made her husband promise to have the doctors executed on her grave if and when she died. Unfortunately for them she did expire, and in agony, and sentence was duly carried out on her grave before the assembled court and in the presence of the other royal physicians, who could scarcely have felt comfortable at watching the spectacle.

Yet, intermixed with this cruelty and barbarism there was an enlightenment in medical manners and mores that seems astonishing to us today. Under Charlemagne, who reigned 768–814, things improved still more, for he took medicine out of the hands of the monks where possible and encouraged young boys to study medical matters. But even before Charlemagne we come across what must be one of the earliest authentic women doctors in the figure of Queen Radegund, who founded a convent and hospital in Poitiers in 570. In view of this it is all the more difficult to understand the attitude of the Victorians and their contemporaries in other countries who so savagely resisted the entry of women into medicine.

It was to be another thirteen hundred years before the first woman was allowed to qualify as a doctor. This was Elizabeth Blackwell (1821–1910) in America, who came from England as a child, and as a young woman stormed the bastions of male-dominated medicine with her two sisters. She finally qualified from the Geneva Medical School of Western New York in 1849 but experienced the greatest difficulty in finding employment in a hospital because of antagonism by the male medical staff. Not to be beaten, in 1850 she opened her own private dispensary for women and children in New York. By the Civil War three medical schools were admitting women as students, though, incredible as it may seem, the Harvard Medical School did not do so until 1945.

In England the situation was very much the same, but, encouraged by Elizabeth Blackwell, an intrepid young woman named Elizabeth Garrett (1836–1917) succeeded in obtaining a medical degree by 1865. By the time her copioneer and friend, Sophia Jex-Blake (1840–1913), had qualified in 1876, the General Medical Council had decided to allow women to practice as doctors, and a law passed that year legalized their position in Britain.

In Christian communities, though the equivalent of the family doctor or general practitioner did not exist, the court physicians, who were nearly always monks, continued to uphold the best medical traditions. Many became famous, like Labeo (thick-lipped) Notker (912–975), a German-Swiss Benedictine of St. Gall, Switzerland, who was also one of the physicians to Duke Henry of Bavaria. When the duke's other medical advisers, jealous of Notker, persuaded the duke to try and catch him out, Henry sent Notker a sample of the urine of a pregnant maid-servant, saying that it was his own. Urine analysis by close study of the color of the liquid when settled was a favorite form of diagnosis from ancient times, and continues to be used in modified form in diabetic and other conditions today. But Notker was not to be fooled so easily. Quickly he made a public announcement to the effect that there would shortly occur the greatest miracle in Christian times—the Duke Henry would be delivered of a child within the next thirty days!

But though men like Notker kept the medical flag flying to the best of their ability, they were not very willing to impart their knowledge to others, and in Europe as a whole the art of scientific healing was deteriorating.

Fortunately it was saved by that curious phenomenon previously mentioned—the survival of Greek language and culture in southern Italy. It was natural that the more erudite scholars of both Europe and the Orient should find a common meeting place in this ambience of ancient culture and learning, and by the ninth century a medical school had been established at Salerno which was to blossom into one of the most famous universities of Europe. Here medical students, teachers, and practitioners from Italy, France, and Germany met their counterparts from Arabia and Persia for an interchange of ideas and a pooling of knowledge that was to have far-reaching results in many spheres, not only medicine.

Much information on medicine in the Near East at the time comes to us from this source, and it is apparent that the period from the tenth to the twelfth century was the golden age of medicine in Arabia. The Arabs were, on the whole, a tolerant race, Jew and Christian being allowed to practice their religion, study medicine, and enter the professions as easily as members of their own race. As noted earlier, the first outstanding Arabian doctor was Rhazes, medical supervisor of the famous hospital in Baghdad. But though medical teaching was at a high level, it did not always percolate down to the ordinary practitioner, where knowledge and ability were very variable. Some took examinations and some did not. The son of a doctor would automatically inherit his father's practice whether or not he showed any skill or aptitude for the work. Due to the death of his son as a result of ill-judged medical treatment, the caliph of Baghdad, in 931, imposed examinations on all those professing to be doctors, exempting only the court physicians and doctors of repute.

This cleanup of the medical profession in Islam was to raise the status of physicians to almost unheard-of heights, and many were later extravagantly paid. Wealthiest of all were the court physicians and "body doctors," the former dealing with internal medicine and the latter specializing in wounds received accidentally or in combat. Both categories were showered with gifts and honors.

In fact the status of the doctor had improved so much that an Arab physician, al-Taburi, could write: "No one should live in any country that does not have four things: a just government, useful medicines, flowing water and an educated physician." This is a long way from the warning to avoid a town where the chief citizen was a physician.

Among the populations of the Near East, Jewish doctors carried on their medical tradition as they had done since Biblical times. Maimonides was probably one of the greatest physicians to emerge from that era, and it is he who is reputed to be the author of that wonderfully humble and reverent supplication to the Almighty known as *The Morning Prayer of the Jewish Physician*.

> Oh God, let my mind be ever clean and enlightened. By the bedside of the patient let no alien thought deflect it. Let everything that experience and scholarship have taught it be present in it, and hinder it not in its tranquil work. For great and noble are

those scientific judgements that serve the purpose of preserving the health and lives of Thy creatures. Keep far from me the delusion that I can accomplish all things. Give me the strength, the will and the opportunity to amplify my knowledge more and more. Today I can disclose things in my knowledge which yesterday I would not yet have dreamt of, for the Art is great, and the human mind presses on untiringly. In the patient let me see ever only the man. Thou, All-Bountiful One, hast chosen me to watch over the life and death of Thy creatures. I prepare myself now for my calling. Stand by me now in this great task, so that it may prosper. For without Thine aid man prospers not even in his smallest dealings.

In Jewish medicine we have another instance of women practicing, if not as fully qualified doctors, in their own specialization of dealing with eye troubles. For many centuries Jewish women were to be honored as the best eye surgeons available, though it was still an era in which the art of the surgeon was considered far inferior to that of the physician.

At Salerno one of the greatest influences at the university was Constantine the African (1015–1089) who came from Carthage. He was an Arab apothecary, and after many years of wandering in Mediterranean countries, he arrived at Salerno in 1065 with a more varied knowledge of drugs and medicine in current use than anyone before. He was a Christian, and after teaching at the university for some years, joined the monastic order at Monte Cassino, not many miles away, where he spent the remainder of his time translating Greek and Arab medical texts into Latin.

Gradually the influence of Salerno, with that of the almost contemporary university of Montpellier, in the south of France, began to be felt throughout Europe as the quest for knowledge began to reassert itself. Other universities gradually became established, notably that of Bologna in 1156, first as a law college, but later veering toward medicine and in particular the art of surgery. The University of Paris also dates from this period, while the next hundred years saw the establishment of universities at Oxford, Cambridge, Naples, and Padua.

Despite this, the progress of medical knowledge among ordinary practitioners was slow, and the major part of those who

attended to the sick in the towns and villages were not in close
touch with teaching at the great universities. The number of
medical students qualifying was small, not usually more than 1
percent of the total number of students. As an example, the city
of Paris in 1292 had only six qualified physicians and, despite the
rise in population, had only ten two centuries later. The mass
of the population was being tended by itinerant quacks or
barber-surgeons, and only the wealthy had the benefits of the
new medical teaching.

Once again an attempt was made to raise the level of knowledge of the ordinary general physician, and in 1140 a new
legal code devised by Roger II, king of Sicily, and authorized by
the pope, contained a section dealing with doctors and their
qualifications. This stipulated that:

> The poor must be treated free.
> A physician should attend for medical examinations after three
> After qualifying he must receive permission to practice from
> years' study of logic and five years' study of medicine.
> the king or his official representative.
> For surgeons, one year of medical studies must be undergone
> and one year's apprenticeship to a qualified surgeon before taking
> the examination.
> Two visits a day must be made if requested by the patient and
> two at night.

Fees for attendance and traveling were laid down, but in
contrast to the code of the Visigoths, no estimate of cost of treatment was to be agreed on beforehand. In addition a division
was established between the duties of the doctor and that of the
apothecary or druggist, for the latter had long been a separate
profession in Eastern medicine. Though these rules were formulated mainly for the benefit of those living around Naples and
the Kingdom of the Two Sicilies, they were found so valuable
that they gradually were adopted in other parts of Italy and in
France and Germany.

By the end of the fourteenth century medical schools as part
of the university had become normal and were an established
fact of the new universities at Heidelberg and Cologne, but the
influence of the Salerno, the forerunner of them all, was begin-

ning to wane. It continued to exist, however, with varying status as a center of learning, until finally closed by an edict of Napoleon in 1811.

In Germany the code was modified, and retained some of the inhuman and cruel treatment that had been reserved for physicians who failed in earlier times. In 1337 a famous eye surgeon of Breslau failed to cure the double vision of King John of Bavaria who, with apparent single-mindedness, had him tossed into the Oder where he drowned.

In France and particularly in the region around Paris there was differentiation between those who had qualified at the university and the ordinary barber-surgeon or wound doctor, the former wearing a long robe and the latter a short one. Even among the surgeons themselves there was strife, the higher grade of university-taught practitioner (of the long robe) being allowed to carry out operations such as brain surgery, removal of intestines and rectal fistules, while those not qualified saw to wounds, bloodletting, hernia operations, the extraction of teeth, and simple bone-setting after fracture.

In England, though the rise in the status of the doctor was slower than in other parts of Europe, there was rivalry between physicians and barber-surgeons from about 1300, a feud which was not resolved for two hundred years when Henry VIII granted separate authorities to each.

But before that happened there occurred in Europe a catastrophe which was to precipitate the most violent antagonism toward doctors ever seen, and to erect a barrier of suspicion and mistrust of medicine that had never been experienced before. It was the Black Death.

The first rumors of a pestilence of epidemic proportions came from the East in 1330 when it was reported that over thirteen million had died in China and that India was depopulated. Gradually the rumors increased as the plague drew nearer to Europe, and soon reports were being received that fifteen thousand a day were dying in Cairo and that not a single man, woman, or child in Cyprus survived.

Needless to say these reports were exaggerated. Travelers

are notorious for their tales, and in the fourteenth century the East was remote and confirmation of facts difficult to obtain. But it was obvious that something was happening, and that it was not only connected with disease. An upheaval in the natural order of things seemed to be going on, confirmed by the eruption of Mount Etna in 1333 and an unprecedented swarm of locusts infesting southern Europe four years later. In 1338 France had its worst harvest ever, in 1342 death and desolation occurred over a wide area when the Rhine burst its banks, and in 1346 comparatively severe earthquakes were felt in northern Italy. Nobody could say why these things were happening, and in the gloom and feeling of imminent disaster that pervaded Europe, there were many who foretold the end of the world.

There were, of course, many Biblical precedents for these phenomena, and it was natural for the population at first to turn to the Church for guidance. There was little comfort to be found there.

As the first deaths in Constantinople were recorded, it became obvious that the plague was soon to ravage Europe. By October of that year it had taken root in Sicily, and by October 1348 had gained a firm hold in northern Italy and France.

The most terrifying aspect of the disease was the speed with which it took its toll. Men and women were struck down as they fled from the town to the country, and no one knew in the morning who would be alive to tell the tale by nightfall. The doctors seemed powerless to stop the progress of the disease, though many theories circulated as to its cause and origin.

In 1348 the physicians of Paris met to discuss the matter and issued a manifesto stating that the plague was due to "cosmic influences" creating a poisonous, damp mist fatal to men, and giving instructions how to combat it. Amongst their instructions were the following:

Do not sleep during the day.
Do not eat cold or moist food.
Do not go out at night.
The consumption of olive oil is fatal.
Bathing is injurious, as is any great exercise, and sexual indulgence is particularly dangerous.

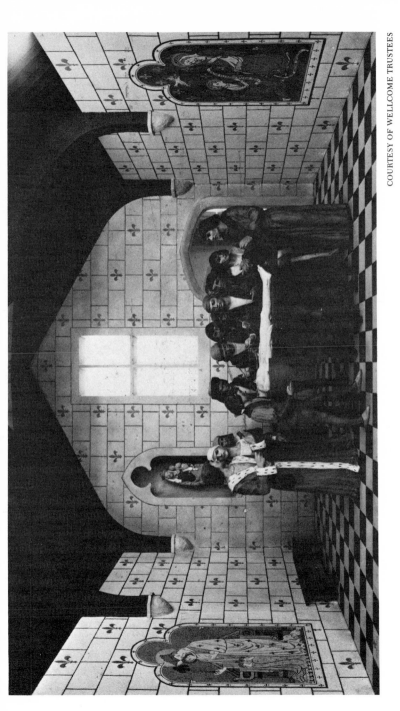

Diorama built for the 1937 Paris Medical Exhibition showing Guy de Chauliac (1300-1370) giving an anatomical demonstration at the University of Montpellier.

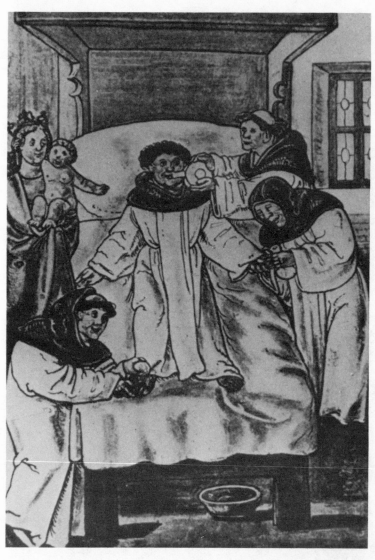

A 1513 Swiss engraving showing the early use of alcohol fumes
as an anesthetic.

They also recommended that a diet of potherbs, such as sage and rosemary, was beneficial, and that a wise precaution was to eat a little treacle after rain. From this it can be seen how sparse was the knowledge of doctors in trying to combat this monumental disaster and how pitiful their precautions.

The Church, on the other hand, went into its normal routine of "disaster as a punishment for sin." It was a standard device and was still much to the fore five hundred years later when the first cholera epidemic hit New York in 1832 and the pastors of the city were to lay the blame on the immigrant Irish Catholic dockers and their "godless" ways.

In the early stages of the Black Death (diagnosed in modern times as three separate forms of bubonic plague), "sin" was equated with "non-Christian," the result being a violent eruption of feeling against the Jews in all European countries. But later, as Church dignitaries themselves fell victim, panic began to take over and the population vented its wrath against the medical profession for its inability to do anything positive.

Not only were the doctors thought to be ignorant, as they largely were, but were also accused of spreading the infection purely for monetary gain, and to be in league with gravediggers and others who appeared to benefit from the calamity. The worst possible combination was to be a Jew and also a doctor. In September 1348 ten Jews, four of them doctors, were tortured mercilessly at the Castle of Chillon, on the Lake of Geneva, and forced to "confess" that they had purposely spread the Black Death and actually murdered wealthy patients. After the most terrible mutilations they were burned to death and their bodies consigned to the lake.

Oddly enough it was their ancient precepts concerning hygiene and health which were to be the Jews' undoing, and seemed to prove their guilt. They recognized that many of the sources of water in use were polluted and potential carriers of the disease, and warned the population to keep away from them. Unfortunately many of the springs and wells were considered holy and associated with miraculous cures, and the advice to keep away from them was considered a sinister plot to spread the infection. There was even a rumor that Jewish doctors in Spain, at the medical school of Toledo, were actually sending poisonous

material to their colleagues in France and Germany in the form
of beetles, spiders, and bats to further their wicked purpose.
The first great massacre of Jews took place in Provence,
France, late in 1348, and similar massacres were soon perpetrated
throughout the land. So grave did the situation become, and so
extraordinary the stories being spread, that the following year
the pope, Clement VI, was forced to publish a bull (that is, a
decree) forbidding attacks on Jews and threatening excommu-
nication for disobedience. It had little effect, and in that terrible
year pogroms were widespread in Mainz, Strasbourg, Basel, and
other cities of Europe, that in Mainz alone being responsible for
the deaths of twelve thousand Jews, many of them doctors. At
Speyer and Eslingen the Jewish population shut themselves in
their houses and burned themselves to death rather than face
death at the hands of the mob, their bodies later being thrown
into the Rhine "to reduce the infection."

In England the Black Death came to a country flushed with
success and riding on the crest of a wave. Edward III's great
victory at Crécy in 1346 had been followed by the capture of
Calais, and, as William of Walsingham was to write later, "A new
sun seemed to have arisen over the people in perfect peace, in
the plenty of all things and in the glory of victories."

It was all the more ironical that it was these very victories
and the great increase in travel between England and the French
Channel ports that should have the effect of bringing the plague
directly to England. By the end of 1349 all the southern counties
of England were in its grip, and chroniclers of the time record
how, in Bristol and in Bath, there were scarce enough living to
bury the dead. Gradually it spread throughout the land, much
to the jubilation of the Scots who considered this God's curse
on their hated enemies, until it struck them woefully in 1350 at
a celebration thanksgiving at Selkirk, where many perished.

In both England and Scotland in those years many tried to
escape by fleeing their homes and going elsewhere. Particularly
prone to do this were the clergy, and some doctors also followed
suit. The majority, however, stayed at their posts to do what they
could, and many succumbed with their patients.

But in Britain as a whole there was never the anti-Jewish

or antidoctor feeling that was such a feature of the plague in other parts of Europe. The doctors who remained at their posts were praised, but for some reason there was great distrust of the nurses who ministered to the sick. More than one incident is recorded of a nurse putting a wet cloth to the face of a patient in an attempt to end his life, though a more charitable explanation may be that it was to end his suffering. The medical profession as a whole, however, was not held in very high regard at that time, and Chaucer's description of the doctor whose garments were "lined with taffata and with sandyl" from the money he made out of "phisick and pestilence" is typical of the general attitude. But a calamity such as this, which is calculated to have killed half the population of Europe, was bound to have serious repercussions on the attitude toward doctors and healing. It was to be two hundred years at least before the medical profession was to recover from the blow.

VII

Anatomists and Surgeons

THOUGH THE EARLY Christian Church had frowned upon the curing of disease by human means as contrary to God's wishes, by the Middle Ages most higher medicine was under the control of the pope and the Vatican. The result of this was mixed. Some papal edicts furthered the cause of healing, others retarded its progress by many years. One of the provisions of the Fourth Lateran Council in 1215, for example, was to prohibit strictly any behavior by the physician which could be thought to endanger the soul of the patient. This included extramarital sexual intercourse, masturbation, alcoholic intoxication, and the breaking of the laws regarding fasting. A code of penalties was established, and though this may well have resulted in a high standard of moral conduct for physicians generally, the benefit of this to the soul of the patient is more problematical.

This same Lateran Council also delayed progress in anatomy and surgery severely by decreeing that no dismemberment of the human body should ever be undertaken for study, and that no physicians should practice amputations or surgery. Conversely, surgeons were also forbidden to do the work of ordinary physicians. This not only created a wide breach between the doctor and the surgeon but made it very difficult for any student of medicine to acquire any knowledge of human anatomy. Few universities taught anatomy, though one of the few to do so was that of Montpellier, in France, where Mondino de' Luzzi (1275–

1326) led an attack against the prohibitions of the Church in this matter. In 1300 a papal decree allowed the occasional dissection (about twice a year) of the corpses of criminals, but for most dissections the bodies of pigs, rhesus monkeys, and Barbary apes were used. Though Mondino (usually called Mundinus) was handicapped by this, he wrote what is usually considered to be the first anatomical textbook of any value, though closely following the teaching of Galen and repeating many of his errors.

It was a pupil of Mundinus, the gifted physician-anatomist Guy de Chauliac (1300–1370) who, in his famous book *Chirurgia magna*, finally brought surgery and anatomy into the light at Avignon, where he was a member of the papal court under Pope Clement VI. There were many who were ready to equate him with Hippocrates in the extent of his learning, which ranged far beyond medicine, and certainly his teaching remained a vital force for the next three hundred years. His ideal of the profession of surgeon was high, and he said: "A good surgeon should be courteous, sober, pious and merciful, not greedy of gain, and with a sense of his own dignity." This was an unusual concept in an era when the majority of those undertaking surgery were unqualified charlatans, classed little better than tradesmen, and his felicity of writing and clarity of expression, together with his very definite and self-assured pronouncements, ensured that his teachings were heeded and discussed.

De Chauliac contracted the plague at the time of the Black Death, recovered from it, and described the symptoms and treatment in another book.

His actions were of importance in that he actually treated ruptures and cataracts of the eye himself, conditions which, at the time, were normally left to the wandering quacks and barber-surgeons. He was also the first physician to use a weighted extension in treating fractures of the leg or arm, and devised the use of a rope over the bed by which the patient could alter his position. He also mentions the use of a narcotic inhalation which enabled operations to be carried out painlessly and was therefore something of a pioneer in the art of anesthesia.

Also at Montpellier at the same time as Guy de Chauliac was an English student, John of Ardern (1307–1390) who, after taking his exams, returned to his native country and practiced as a surgeon, traveling constantly between Nottingham and London. He was a specialist in diseases of the lower bowel and invented a new operation for anal fistula. He recognized and described cancer of the rectum, warning that no operation could be successful and that the patient would surely die. Typical of his times, however, his teaching and treatment were a mixture of science and magicoreligious ritual, such as his recommended cure for piles: to write the names of the Trinity on paper with the blood from the little finger, and say three Paternosters.

In the middle of the fifteenth century and the beginning of the sixteenth, two events took place which had a profound effect on the dissemination of medical knowledge and also created an entirely new concept of treatment. One was the invention of printing from movable type by Gutenberg about 1450, the other the rise of a man who was to make himself famous as a fighter for medical reform—Theophrastus Bombastus von Hohenheim, better known as Paracelsus (1493–1541).

The advent of printing allowed the works of Galen, Avicenna, Mundinus, and others to be read more widely and their theories discussed. Paracelsus was one who disagreed violently with most of them.

He was born in Switzerland and was the son of a country doctor practicing near Zurich. During his formative years he accompanied his father on his visits, often to the lead mines at Fugger, where his interest in mineralogy was first aroused. He qualified as a doctor, probably at Basel, and then traveled extensively, first in England, where he visited the tin mines of Cornwall, and then to France, Spain, Germany, Italy, Turkey, and eventually Russia. In 1526 he returned to Switzerland and was appointed town physician of Basel and professor of medicine at the university there.

All during his travels he had been observing, formulating new ideas and writing them down. As soon as he began teaching at the university the unexpected turn of some of his theories began to be felt, and immediately he was the center of discussion and argument.

He was violently opposed to the practice of surgery and also believed that the human body was composed basically of three elements—sulfur, mercury, and salt. The practice of medicine, he maintained, should be founded on the four pillars of philosophy, astronomy, alchemy, and virtue, of which philosophy was the most important. Anyone entering the profession by any other means was a criminal and a knave. Needless to say, theories such as these brought him into instant conflict with the more reactionary elements of the university, and his notoriety reached new heights when he prefaced a course of lectures by publicly burning the works of Galen. "My shoe buckles are more learned than Galen," he announced in a characteristic burst of modesty, "and my beard knows more than any ancient writer."

Even his belief in astronomy as an adjunct of medicine was not in conformity with the accepted view, for he did not believe in horoscopes nor that the stars controlled man's destiny. Alchemy, he considered, was a most important subject for study, as was a good knowledge of metallurgy, for this enabled poisons to be extracted from foods to the benefit of the patient. He was also an ardent believer in the "doctrine of signatures," that ancient idea that "like cured like." The lungs of a fox, for example, were a specific for bronchitis. The cyclamen, with its ear-shaped leaf, was a cure for deafness, and the little eyebright, from its appearance, could alleviate failing sight. It is a concept that is deeply rooted in medical folklore, and even survives today in rural communities.

Paracelsus also had a curious belief in the existence of a "magic" wound salve which could cure the wound by being applied to the weapon which had caused it, another ancient idea which was to be revived yet again by Sir Kenelm Digby in England in the seventeenth century.

All these strange theories were enunciated by the physician during his professorship at Basel, where he was the first teacher to lecture in German instead of the mandatory Latin which, he said, was merely a cloak for ignorance. Needless to say his outspoken comments and his rantings against the establishment made it impossible for his appointment to be continued, and he was forced to resign. He continued traveling, teaching, and writing and died at Salzburg in 1541.

Whatever one thinks of the ideas and teachings of Paracelsus, he was certainly a character and an original. He stimulated new thoughts about medicine, contributed significantly to pharmacology and to the art of dispensing, and demonstrated the medicinal value of many metallic elements, including the salts of iron and antimony. Alcoholic and syphilitic he might have been (as many of his contemporaries insisted), but he was undoubtedly honest and sincere in all he taught. As he himself forecast, he continued to be misunderstood for many years after his death, but still remains one of the most enigmatic and entertaining figures in medical history. His attitude can best be summed up in his own comment: "I pleased nobody except the people I cured."

Three years before the death of Paracelsus a young Flemish physician was appointed to the chair of anatomy and surgery at the University of Padua, Italy. He was Andreas Vesalius (1514–1564), later to be hailed as the father of modern anatomy. Vesalius was twenty-three when he took up his appointment. He came from a family of doctors and apothecaries and at an early age displayed an interest in the dissection of small animals such as birds and mice. As a surgeon he, too, was frustrated by the difficulties of finding sufficient human bodies to dissect, for this was still considered unethical if not downright blasphemous, and he was conscious of the effect this had had on the anatomical teachings of Galen, with which he disagreed.

He determined to investigate the human body and disregard the ethics of the matter, and published his findings in a most sumptuous and important book called *De Humani Corporis Fabrica* (On the Fabric of the Human Body), published in 1543. The anatomical plates which adorned the book, probably by Jan Stevenszoon van Calcar, were the finest ever seen and have served as models for generations of medical students ever since.

The book begins with a lament for the decline of the art of healing. Surgery, bleeding, and cupping, he says, are left to the itinerant barbers, dietetic matters to the cooks. He is at his most bitter when describing the teaching of anatomy in medical schools:

The deplorable method of instruction which is used today demands that one person—generally a surgeon or a barber—should carry out the dissection of the human body, while the lecturer reads a description of the different parts of the body derived from books. While he does so he sits enthroned on his rostrum and, with looks of obvious disdain, he expounds hypotheses on facts which he can in no way know from his own experience, but which he has learned by heart from the books of others or which he has just read from the book that lies before him. Those who are actually performing the dissection are so ignorant that they are in fact not in a position to demonstrate to the students the parts which they are preparing, or to explain them, and as the professor never touches the body and as the dissector does not know the Latin names and therefore cannot follow the lecture in sequence, each goes his own way. Hence the instruction is very bad, days are lost dealing with silly questions, and in the confusion the student learns less than a butcher could teach the professor.

Vesalius determined to rectify this state of affairs by doing the dissections himself, and in the process corrected many of the errors and misconceptions propagated by Galen. He showed that the sternum, or breastbone, was composed of three parts, not seven. He demonstrated the true shape of the liver and of the uterus, and drew attention to the valves in the veins, though he did not appreciate their true function. What created a major sensation was his demolition of the age-old fable dating from the Old Testament that men had one rib fewer than women.

There were many who listened to Vesalius with disquiet, considering that to doubt the teaching of Galen was compounding a heresy, and there were others who fiercely opposed him. When he showed that the hipbone in man was far more narrow than Galen had thought, his opponents claimed that Galen had been right in his day, but that the male hipbone had become constricted since by the habit of wearing tight breeches! Like Paracelsus before him, Vesalius finally resigned his tutorial chair and traveled abroad, continuing to teach and write. He eventually died in a shipwreck off the Gulf of Corinth on his way back from a pilgrimage to the Holy Land.

Unlike Paracelsus, however, Vesalius was soon vindicated as anatomical research went forward with more knowledge and fewer restrictions.

The period immediately following Vesalius produced surgeons whose names are forever perpetuated in anatomical nomenclature.

Gabriel Fallopius (1523–1562), for example, was an eminent researcher whose discovery of the Fallopian tubes of the uterus marked a turning point in gynecology. Another was Bartholomeus Eustachius (1524?–1574) who has given his name to the balancing canals of the ear.

But it was a humble barber-surgeon who was destined to act on the teachings of Vesalius and to go far in making surgery an honorable profession. He was the Frenchman, Ambroise Paré (1510–1590), a man destined to be one of the most famous surgeons of all time.

The reason for his rise to prominence rests largely on the invention of gunpowder and the infliction of a new type of wound, and the fact that for many years he was a wound surgeon in the army. His anatomical knowledge and surgical skill were such that during the thirty years he followed the armies and tended the wounded, his fame rose to the extent that, before the end of his long life, he succeeded in being surgeon to four kings of France in succession. Although he knew no Latin and had received no formal education, he was appointed to the chair of anatomy at the University of Paris, and after his brilliant army career spent many years teaching and acting as a court physician. He invented many surgical instruments which are still in use today, and revolutionized the treatment of fractures and gunshot wounds.

In England, though the status of the barber-surgeon had been slowly rising, there were few writers (with the exception of John of Ardern) who have left an accurate account of the exact standing of the trade. It is known that since the fourteenth century the English barber-surgeons had been forming themselves into loose guilds based in the larger towns, but in 1540 they finally achieved improved status and royal recognition. In that year an act of Henry VIII established the official City Livery Company of Barber-Surgeons with its own laws, its four masters (two being barbers and two surgeons) and, like most livery companies, a seven-year apprenticeship before being allowed full membership.

In Scotland similar status was given to the barber-surgeons a little later, with the curious and valuable advantage that they were given the sole right for the distillation of whiskey in any town in which they were represented.

For two hundred years the barbers and surgeons of Britain acted in concert through their Livery Company until they were finally separated in 1745, the medical side of the company developing later into the Royal College of Surgeons, still the governing body of the profession in Britain today.

The practice of surgery and anatomy in the United States of America suffered from the same opposition to dissection that had hampered it for so many years in Europe. Among the first students the study of anatomy was difficult owing to the sparse population and the absence of suitable corpses, but according to Judge Samuel Stillwell, writing in 1676, there was no objection to the dissection of the bodies of Indians. Nearly a hundred years later a month's course in dissection for medical students was offered by a surgeon, Thomas Wood, in New York and was advertised by the New York *Weekly Postboy* in January 1752. In 1765 the University of Philadelphia officially took over the anatomical course begun as a private enterprise by Dr. William Shippen (1736–1808), a well-known army surgeon and later founder of the College of Physicians of Philadelphia.

Unfortunately, as happened in Britain, the public reacted violently to what they considered a flagrant disregard of what was ethically correct, particularly as rumors soon spread that graves were being violated and cadavers stolen for the progress of anatomical research. It was useless for the surgeons to insist that only bodies of criminals and suicides were being used, and the matter eventually came to a head in the riots known as the Doctors Mob in New York in 1788. This was sparked off by a misguided sense of humor on the part of a surgeon who, seeing a small boy peering through the window of the dissecting room, cheerfully waved the leg of a corpse at him in greeting. The terrified boy repeated a garbled and highly colored account of the incident, which was seized on by a mob who finally attacked the laboratory. The medical staff took refuge in the local jail, which was attacked by the mob in turn. Not until the militia was summoned and seven rioters killed did things quiet down.

In 1798 the New York Assembly officially authorized the dissection of the bodies of those convicted of arson, burglary, and murder, and gradually other states followed suit. In 1831 Massachusetts extended the law to cover "all deceased persons buried at the publick expense."

One of the reasons for the unrest and misgivings on the part of the public was that rumors of body snatching from graves were not without foundation. Surgeons short of bodies were not likely to ask too many questions when accepting delivery of a corpse. The business was in the hands of the notorius "resurrection men," and it was well known that many surgeons, if not taking an active part in the process, certainly condoned it and in some cases instigated it. The following graphic description of one such raid is provided by John Knyveton, a London medical student, in 1752.

> January 5.: Was up again all last night Corpse Taking. Would have performed the task on the evening of Jan 3 only Mr.St.Clair had that night to dine with his father, and the new graveyard being a good mile from Dr.Urquhart's we did need all our company. As before, the doctor did lend us his Man, but would know nothing of our doings: and after some discussion we did deem it wise to recruit our numbers, as the streets we were to traverse are roamed at nights by Footpads and Bully Boys. So at the Infirmary that day we did gather the Class together and disclosed to them our Plans; at which they did all want to come, but we made them draw lots thus selecting four and by God's grace did get the most lusty crew. And so to gather at the Doctor's, and at half after midnight out into the roads and down to the river; catching a glimpse of two lots of Gentlemen of the Road but they not molesting us from the quantity of our numbers. Dr.Urquhart's Servant did take our bringing extra numbers but ill, asking us why we did not bring some chairmen with torches and a fife and drum; but to calm him with a guinea and he grumbling to lead the way. The night was very dark and bitter cold and the streets thereby empty for which we were very grateful. The graveyard surrounded by a Very High Wall entered by an Iron Gate, which was locked. At which we were all dismayed, but the Huge Serving Man did produce a master key and so we did gain entrance.
>
> The graveyard was a large one, but we had marked the site of the grave and so found our way to it with tolerable ease, one of the Young Men however catching his knee against a Tomb Stone

and severely bruising his Patella or Knee Pan, at which he did swear lustily. Then to dig, and by our numbers soon to uncover the coffin; and so to burst it open and drag out the body within, this being a man of some forty years, very well developed, at which we were well pleased. Then to drag off his shroud, and the moon comes out faint from behind a cloud and shines on us, at which one Young Gentleman near took Hystericks; the more so as the Doctor's man drops his spade with a great clatter and cries out with a Fearful Oath that it was his cousin, who had, it seems, been a Highwayman but lately caught and hanged, Dr.Urquhart's servant knowing nothing of this. So we to stuff the body in the Sack, he muttering away beneath his breath; and so with some relief of Spirits out into the Lane again. There we did have the misfortune to find some Bully Boys awaiting us, they passing and hearing the noise when the Body was Stripped. They did set upon us with loud cries and I being one of the foremost was straightway beaten down into the gutter, where George Blumenfeld him in a minute join me, and I very wroth and thankful that we were in force that we might teach those Bullies and Virgin-Breakers a Lesson. So the fight was joined and I to my feet did tug out my Small Sword and to my great satisfaction did receive the rush of one upon its point so his arm was pierced, the which was a lesson to me how soft the flesh be during life, when not stiffened by that Coagulation of the Humours called Rigor Mortis. There were I suppose some half dozen of them and the fight did rage right heartily until Dr.Urquhart's man forced his way into the press, and taking two of the young bucks by the throat, did knock their heads together with such force that they were stunned, and so the rest took to their heels and we in triumph with the corpse to Dr.Urquhart's where as heretofore I did pass the night on the couch.

The same year as young Knyveton was involved in this grisly incident came the first authenticated case of a murder being committed to provide a suitable corpse for the surgeons. This had been perpetrated by two nurses, females of a very low type as were most nurses in the eighteenth century, who had taken a mother and her child, plied them with drink and suffocated them. Both women were convicted and hanged, but still many others were prepared to take the risk. The most famous of these were the infamous Edinburgh body snatchers, William Burke and William Hare, who during 1827 and 1828 were in partnership as resurrection men and were thought to have accounted for the death of at least sixteen men and women, the bodies of all of whom were sold to a Dr. James Knox, who conducted a school of anatomy. After their arrest, Hare turned king's evidence and Burke was duly convicted. Dr. Knox, though technically innocent, was forced to leave town hurriedly to avoid the enraged mob, and William Burke was hanged publicly in Edinburgh before a crowd of thirty thousand on January 29, 1829.

The result of the Burke and Hare case was the passing of new laws in both Britain and America controlling the supply of corpses to medical schools.

That our surgical and anatomical knowledge is so complete today is due to a very large extent to the work of the early anatomists, carrying out their task against formidable odds and even in this century still encountering opposition. This happened in 1901 in Chicago, when John Alexander Dowie, leader of a new religious sect, began a violent program of scaremongering based on the grounds that corpses used for dissections might not, in fact, be dead.

Difficulties still existed well into the nineteenth century, however, and unimpeded progress in surgical techniques could not really develop until the coming of anesthetics and the evolution of antisepsis.

These two factors ensured the progress of medical research, and in time gave rise to a long line of eminent surgeons, both in Europe and America, who will be dealt with in a later chapter.

VIII

Quack Doctors and Impostors

ONE OF THE PROBLEMS that has always been inherent in medical legislation and the protection of health is that, while the very poor are safeguarded and the rich can pay for themselves, little regard is given to the lot of the low-paid worker. The free treatment available to the pauper is not for him, by reason of his earnings, yet he cannot afford the charges of the legitimate physician.

It was so in Greek and Roman times and was certainly true in seventeenth-century Europe. The result, in both periods, was for the poor and uneducated laborer to resort to magical or quasi-religious devices, and to quacks and charlatans, in effort to gain a cheap cure.

In Britain, during Cromwell's day, quack medicine was sparse and virtually underground, being confined mainly to itinerant herbalists and pseudodoctors and dentists attending country fairs and markets. But the restoration of Charles II in 1660 opened the floodgates, and the quack came into his own. Many such had been on the fringe of the royal court in Europe, and accompanied the court back to England with spurious claims of a royal appointment. But the relaxed and more permissive climate of the times provided a breeding ground for quackery of every kind, and anyone with even the most elementary medical knowledge set about making his fortune.

In America, due perhaps to the puritanical background of the early settlers, the phenomenon of the quack did not occur so soon. The settlers brought some primitive forms of medication with them, of course, but very early on found themselves using the herbal preparations of the native Indians. These, like a great deal of folk medicine, were based very much more on science and observation than was fully realized, and mostly did the job for which they were employed.

The settlers noted how the Delaware and Iroquois Indians used the leaves of the foxglove for heart conditions, and, later, how in the upper Mississippi, comfrey plants served as an antidote for burns and bruises. Among most tribes tobacco, either chewed or smoked, served as a panacea for a variety of ills and in powder form was a cure for wounds and injuries.

But in the Old World more commercial, yet far less successful forms of therapy were coming into vogue. Both in the form of treatment and in medication, the late seventeenth century and particularly the eighteenth century were the golden age of quackery.

Yet, before looking at some of these charlatans and their nostrums, let us consider just what is meant by a "quack" remedy. Even the derivation of the word is uncertain. It probably stems from "quacksalver," from the Dutch *kwaksalver*, to boast of one's salves. Others consider it comes from the fact that medicinemen "quacked" their wares about the marketplaces like ducks, or from the vogue for the mercury quicksilver, or "quacksilver," in medicine that was such a feature of the seventeenth century. But whatever the etymology, it is normally reserved either for a medicine of no value at all, or for the man who sold it. Yet in the light of our present-day knowledge of the action of placebos, we know that even an apparently useless drug *can* exert a beneficial effect if the patient really has faith in it and thinks that it will work. It would also be a mistake to think that this applies to only very guillible and not very intelligent people. Dr. Henry K. Beecher, of Harvard, has conducted many experiments on the action of placebos in such instances as postoperative pain, angina, coughs, headaches, and seasickness and has demonstrated that guillibility and intelligence have very little to do with the effect claimed. With every placebo used, about 15 percent of the patients are certain that it is giving relief, the extraordinary thing being that the condition claimed is often measurable. Temperatures actually do drop, coughs dry up, the heart beats more regularly, and headaches disappear, yet no drug of any value has been used on the patient. Nobody so far has been able to explain this phenomenon.

The question of quackery, therefore, must be approached with an open mind and we should not be too quick to condemn. Many forms of treatment, if they depart from what is expected, have been looked upon as quackery, if not ascribed to the intervention of the devil himself. There are numerous instances of this in medical history.

In 1552 Geronimo Cardano (1501–1576), a famous physician of the University of Padua, was summoned to Edinburgh in the hope that he would be able to relieve the Scottish Archbishop Hamilton of asthma. His method of treatment, which consisted of introducing a Spartan regime into the archbishop's life-style, ensuring plenty of exercise and fresh air and banning his custom of having a woman every night before and after supper, seems commonsensical enough today. And it worked, though the archbishop's own physicians accused Cardano of witchcraft and black magic. Fortunately this was not the view of the archbishop himself who, in gratitude to the Italian, paid him handsomely and begged him to call on him "in any circumstances that give trouble." Cardano does not seem to have taken the archbishop up on this, for troubles he had in plenty when he returned to Italy and found his many successes in healing had bred envy and spite among his contemporaries. His cure of a woman with tuberculosis, by sending her to live in the mountains of Switzerland, precipitated an accusation of dealing with the powers of darkness. With evidence against him largely provided by his children, this brilliant doctor was finally thrown into jail where his mind gave way. After some years he was released, recovered his sanity, and devoted the remainder of his life to treating the poor free of charge.

It is a sad commentary that Cardano, in common with many other brilliant physicians whose ideas were eventually proved right, should be looked upon as charlatans while many obvious quacks and impostors achieved fame and fortune. But this has always been so, particularly in medicine, where the more bizarre and unlikely the treatment, the more it is accepted as the wonder cure of the age.

Not surprisingly, many of the quack remedies and philters sold were devoted to the pursuit of love and many claimed to have aphrodisiacal powers. All the great herbals of the age have listed plants specially suitable for that purpose, and include:

> Carrot—a powerful aphrodisiac allowing one to see in the dark
> Fern seed—the spores give men power over women
> Cyclamen—a good "amorous" medicine

Many quacks made a specialty of dealing with love potions, and made fortunes as a result, as did "Dr." Thomas Tennant, a notorious London quack in the reign of Charles I who once managed to obtain twenty dollars for a single love philter. Though Tennant was undoubtedly a quack, it would be unfair to stigmatize all those who sold peculiar remedies by this name. Many of those who proffered treatment were quite convinced that it would work, and this fact should distinguish them from the real quacks. Paracelsus himself was described as a quack in the seventeenth century, yet nobody could have believed more implicitly in his own teachings. The true quack is one who knows his treatment is valueless, but still sings its praises and attempts to make money out of it. And there are certainly plenty of these in medical history.

One of the best-known instances of a quack remedy sold for a considerable sum was, in fact, the famous English Drops marketed by a legitimate physician, Dr. Goddard, in the reign of Charles II. The good doctor promoted these drops (later known as Goddard's Drops) as a cure for everything from the common cold to smallpox and syphilis, and succeeded in selling to the British Government the "secret" formula for fifteen thousand dollars. The drops proved to be nothing more than aromatic spirits of ammonia (the active ingredient of smelling salts), the doubtful value of which must have been known to the doctor. This is a good example of the thin borderline between the quack and the legitimate physician, for here we have a respectable and qualified physician selling what was undoubtedly a quack rem-

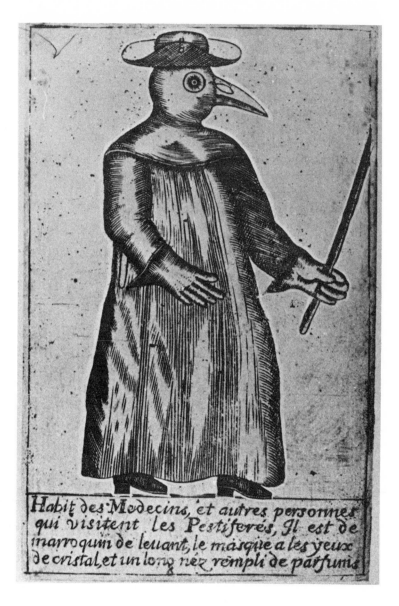

Habit des Medecins, et autres personnes
qui visitent les Pestiferés, Il est de
marroquin de levant, le masque a les yeux
de cristal, et un long nez rempli de parfums

A doctor dressed for treating plague patients in 1656. The beak-like
nosepiece is filled with fragrant herbs to ward off infection
and to mask the smell.

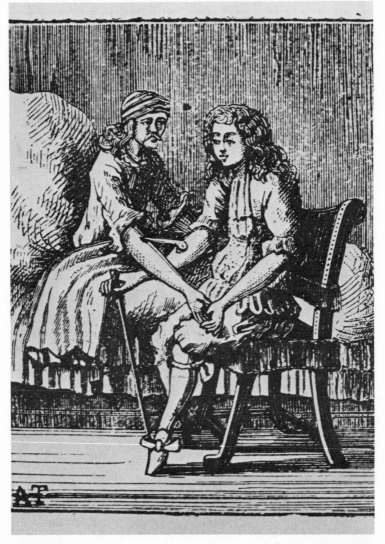

An early attempt at human blood transfusion from a medical book
published in Nuremberg in 1679.

edy, while many so-called quacks were selling herbal concoctions which actually did a certain amount of good.

Fifty years or so after Goddard a woman quack, Joanna Stevens, claimed to have a secret cure for "the stone," which she offered to sell to the government for ten thousand dollars. The subscription list was headed by the duke of Richmond and various gullible clergymen, but after six months the total sum subscribed had reached only four thousand dollars. Incredible as it may seem, the government authorized the balance to be made up from public funds, and the remedy was purchased. In any event the formula was found to be mainly chalk, eggshells, coltsfoot, and carrot seeds in a mixture of soap and honey. Joanna took her ten thousand dollars and was never heard of again.

In 1685 an ingenious gentleman of Maiden Lane, in London, safeguarded himself by advertising a product claiming to protect from several disorders "as yet unknown to the world." These included "The Strong Fives, the Wambling Trot, the Marthambles, the Moon-Fall and the Hockogrockle." As no patient ever contracted these diseases, for they did not exist, the seller was presumably safe in claiming 100 percent success for his product.

The success of the quack doctor in eighteenth-century England is all the more remarkable when one looks at the terrifying list of ingredients used. Nobody, unless he was quite certain he was ill, would willingly have swallowed mixtures which included Red Coral, Crab's Claws, Calcined Human Bones and Grease from a Hanged Man's Scalp, to say nothing of Live Toads, Powdered Earthworms, and Goose Dung. Most of these ingredients were invoked either as part of the doctrine of signatures or as a relic of the "filth therapy" of ancient times by which it was believed that disgusting and repellent medicines would nauseate the malevolent spirits, causing the disease and so drive them away. King James of Scotland, an expert on spirits and exorcism, and author of a best-seller on witchcraft, was convinced that the best method of driving out a devil was the use of tobacco smoke.

The Great Plague which ravaged London in 1665 provided a wonderful opportunity for the countless quacks who thronged the malevolent spirits causing the disease and so drive them by the score, selling amulets of quicksilver to be worn around the neck, infusions of dried mistletoe and the inevitable "dung possets" and mixtures containing "mummy flesh." One of the most incredible prescriptions sold was as follows:

> Take the brains of a young man that hath died a violent death, together with its membranes, arteries, veins, nerves and all the pith of the backbone: bruise these in a stone mortar until it becomes a kind of pap, then put in as much spirits of wine as will cover three fingers breadths, digest for half a year in horse-dung, and take a drop or two in water once a day.

Apart from the fact that this was a rather long-term remedy for anyone suffering from the plague, the chances of actually getting the prescription filled must have been remote. Yet people are known to have bought this prescription in quantity, as they did another specific called "The Countess of Kent's Powder" which contained (or so it was stated) the black extremities of crabs' feet, pearls, the venom of vipers, and a stag's heart. It was guaranteed to "strengthen the heart and all the noble parts" and to cure smallpox, bubonic plague, and measles. One noted quack, the impudent Dr. Case, was honest enough to state on an advertising leaflet:

> *Read, judge and Try,*
> *And if you Die,*
> *Never believe me More!*

But Dr. Case and his colleagues were small fry compared with the success achieved by Ned Ward between 1730 and 1761. Ned (usually called "Spot" Ward because of a birthmark on his face) began his business career running a drysalting business in the City of London in the early 1700s. In 1716 he tried to get into Parliament, believing he was destined for greater things, and was apparently elected as Member for the town of Marlborough in Wiltshire. Investigations soon revealed an extraordinary state of affairs whereby Ward, in collusion with a bribed election official, had managed to get himself elected without a single vote being cast in his favor. As a result of the scandal Ward had to flee to France, where he lived in the area of Dunkirk for the next sixteen years, and worked as an assistant to an apothecary, experimenting with his own pills and potions.

In 1733 he returned to England (having first obtained a free pardon from King George II) and established himself as a "doctor" in London. By great good fortune he was successful in obtaining several much-publicized cures, and his drops and pills became much sought after among the aristocracy, whom he cultivated. Both drops and pills consisted mainly of antimony, a highly toxic substance which could cause violent stomach upsets. Yet the public flocked to buy them, and the occasional demise of a patient after taking the cure did nothing to diminish Ward's status. But his greatest stroke of luck was happening to be in the vicinity when the corpulent king stumbled on a cobblestone, and, putting out his hand to save himself, dislocated his thumb. Ward dexterously wrenched it back into position, and the king, after first kicking him in the shins in his agony, was so impressed that he gave Ward a carriage and pair and allowed him the privilege of driving in the royal parks in London. After that there was no stopping him and when, in 1748, the Apothecaries Act banned all unlicensed practitioners from compounding medicine, Ward was specifically exempted though he had no qualifications of any kind.

He made a fortune during his long life, and in old age gave away considerable sums to charity and treated the poor free. He contributed a sum of two hundred dollars to the citizens of Boston, after "the late dreadful fire" of 1760. At his death in 1761 he was found to be worth about fifty thousand dollars and to own four large houses in the West End of London. Good going for a quack of whom the rhymesters once said:

> Before you take his Drop or Pill
> Take leave of friends and make your will.

Another highly successful quack, but one who made his fortune through clever advertising, was William Brodum. His first ventures into medical quackery were mild enough until he wrote his famous two-volume book called *A Guide to Old Age and a Cure for the Indiscretions of Youth*. It was the "cure" part of the book, contained in the second volume, that brought him notoriety. Brodum said in his introduction, "to Youths I Write and Virgins Uninformed," but any virgin reading the work was not likely to remain uninformed for long.

Brodum blazed the trail for the sexual quackery that was to

reach such vast proportions in nineteenth-century America, and
was the first to cash in on cures for "unnatural vice" and "pernicious practices."

Brodum obtained his qualification as a physician in 1791 from
the two-hundred-year-old Marischal College of the University of
Aberdeen, a curious and slightly bogus institution that handed
out medical diplomas for cash without the necessity of an examination or even an interview. Normally the diploma was accepted
by the Royal College of Physicians in London, but when Brodum
began advertising his sexual cures they felt things had gone too
far and attempted to withdraw his license. It was then found
that because of the way its constitution had been worded, it was
impossible for the Marischal College to cancel its diploma, so the
Royal College of Physicians had to content itself with issuing
stern warnings to patients against the advertisements and activities
of Dr. Brodum, as he was now permitted to call himself. They
were singularly unsuccessful, for Brodum's advertising was force-
ful and potent, even by present-day standards. He was the first
to sell mixtures in several sizes, including a family size that contained five times the quantity in the standard bottle, for only
four times the price.

The claims made by Brodum for his medicines would have
been impressive if true. Apart from luckless victims of masturbation who were saved from the worst and put back on the right
path, he also claimed to have cured a man whose limbs had been
paralyzed for six years. One of his most successful advertisements was for his "Social Happiness Cordial" which, when taken
by married couples, ensured long life, health, and happiness for
their offspring.

Brodum duly retired from the scene, but his place was taken
by other, if less imaginative quacks, who made a nonstop
procession during the late eighteenth and early nineteenth centuries. There was the notorious "Doctor Katterfelto" (it was, in
fact, his name) who gave demonstrations in London and lectured
on mathematics, optics, magnetism, electricity, astronomy, "styan-
graphy, and the palenchic and caprimantic arts," the last all
being subjects of his own invention.

There was Dr. James, whose powders cured fevers of every

kind, including "Intermittent, Remittent, Inflammatory, Nervous, Purple, Yellow or Putrid." By great good fortune the powders were taken up by John Newbury, a London bookseller, who in 1760 was laying the foundations of the wholesale drug business that was later developed by his son, Francis Newbury, so successfully that it was to serve the pharmacists of Britain for the next two hundred years. Dr. James's Fever Powders became a byword as a result, and the writer Oliver Goldsmith is said to have died directly as a result of taking excess quantities of Powders for the Purple Fever.

A later eighteenth-century quack doctor was James Graham, who qualified at Edinburgh in 1770. He went to America and was a successful practitioner in Philadelphia until 1778. In 1779 he moved to Paris where he renewed acquaintance with Benjamin Franklin whom he had previously met in America.

In 1780 he took up residence in London and published various books drawing attention to himself and to the new electrical treatment he was giving. These were conducted in his "Temple of Health and Hymen" just off the Strand in London. At the Temple he employed several beautiful young girls who sang and danced in flimsy costumes, the doctor's contention being that illness could be cured only in the presence of beautiful sights and sounds. It is of interest that one of these young girls, all of whom were said to be virgins, was sixteen-year-old Emma Lyon, later to find a place in history as Emma, Lady Hamilton, Nelson's mistress.

But Graham's pièce de résistance was his gigantic Celestial and Magentico-Electrico bed which could be hired by childless couples at $250 a night with the guarantee that the wife would become pregnant even if she had hitherto been infertile. By all accounts the bed was an incredible sight and is said to have cost the doctor $2500. It might be as well to let Graham describe it in his own words:

> The Grand Celestial Bed, whose magical influences are now celebrated from pole to pole and from the rising to the setting of the sun, is 12ft. long by 9 ft.wide, supported by forty pillars of brilliant glass of the most exquisite workmanship, in richly variegated colours. The super-celestial dome of the bed, which contains

the odoriferous, balmy and ethereal spices, odors and essences, which is the grand reservoir of those reviving invigorating influences which are exhaled by the breath of the music and by the exhilarating force of the electric fire, is covered on the other side with brilliant panes of looking-glass.

On the utmost summit of the dome are placed two figures, Cupid and Psyche, with a figure of Hymen behind with his torch a celestial crown, sparkling over a pair of living turtle doves on a little bed of roses.

The other elegant group of figures which sport on the top of the dome, having each of them musical instruments in their hands, which by the most expensive mechanism, breathe forth sound corresponding to their instruments, flutes, guitars, violins, clarinets, trumpets, horns, oboes, kettle drums etc.

At the head of the bed appears sparkling with electric fire a great first commandment, 'BE FRUITFUL, MULTIPLY AND REPLENISH THE EARTH'. Under that is an excellent sweet-toned organ in front of which is a fine landscape of moving figures, priest and bride's procession entering the Temple of Hymen.

In the Celestial Bed no feather is employed but mattresses filled with sweet new wheat or oat straw mingled with balm, rose leaves, lavender flowers and oriental spices. The sheets are of the richest and softest silks, stained of various colours, and suited to the complexion. Pale green, rose colour, sky blue, white and purple, and are sweetly perfumed in oriental manner with the tudor rose, or with rich gums or balsam.

The chief principle of my Celestial Bed is produced by artificial lodestones. About 15cwt. of compound magnets are continually pouring forth an everflowing circle.

The bed is constructed with a double frame, which moves on an axis or pivot and can be converted to any inclined plane.

Some of the mattresses are filled with the strongest, most springy hair, produced at vast expense from the tails of English stallions which are elastic to the highest degree.

The bed, as can be seen, was a curious mixture of "modern" science and magic. The fact that it could tilt no doubt made it more possible for the male sperm to impregnate the female, while the stallion hairs were a relic of the doctrine of signatures, stallions being famous in song and story for their power to propagate. "Superior ecstasy," said Graham, "which the parties enjoy in the Celestial Bed is really astonishing and never before thought of in this world. The barren must certainly become fruitful when they are powerfully agitated in the delights of love."

Graham did exceedingly well with his bed for a year or two, but the novelty began to fail and he removed to a less fashionable address, presumably to reduce his overhead expenses. But things never came back to their original state, and Graham was eventually reduced to eking out his income with supplying false teeth and a patent dentifrice. He also engaged in a violent bout of propaganda against fornication and masturbation and wrote pamphlet after pamphlet on the subject with strong religious undertones which seemed to presage the religious mania which was finally to overcome him. At the same time he had some sound ideas for encouraging matrimony among the lower classes (who could rarely afford it in the eighteenth century) and suggested a tax on bachelors and spinsters and a bonus for the first child born in wedlock.

He eventually dismantled his Celestial Bed and turned his attention to a new curative process—earth bathing. In this his patients were buried up to the neck in soil while "ethereal balsams" were wafted in their direction. This was not a popular treatment for long, and at the end Graham retired to Edinburgh, where he plunged into a fervor of antisex religiosity and finally died in 1794 from a cerebral hemorrhage.

Perhaps the most elegant quack who ever lived, and certainly one of the most famous, was John St. John Long, who flourished in London in the first quarter of the nineteenth century. He was born in Ireland in 1798 and came to London as a young man. As the result of some elementary art training in Dublin he became assistant to the famous portrait painter, Sir Thomas Lawrence (though there are some who say his assistance took the form of merely cleaning out the great man's studio). What is certainly true is that Long soon acquired a talent for anatomical drawings, which he was able to sell to the various medical schools in London, and so developed an interest in medicine. He decided to set himself up as healer, and by the time he was thirty had become so well-known in this field that he found he could give up art for good.

Dark, dandified, and very good-looking, Long was extremely popular with the ladies, yet never in the whole of his career was a breath of scandal attached to his name. He was charming and gracious, and there is no doubt that part of his extraordinary success was due in no small measure to his native Irish blarney.

He decided to specialize in tuberculosis, a disease which, in the early nineteenth century, was extremely common and carried off a depressingly large number of young people. Long claimed to have invented a liniment which, if rubbed on the patient's body, would "draw out" the disease leaving a telltale area of red as a sign. If the skin showed no reaction the disease was not present.

Once tuberculosis had been diagnosed, special inhalations were provided and the patch of inflamed skin treated by the application of raw cabbage leaves.

There was no shortage of clients and Long soon had a set of offices in Fitzroy Square, in London's West End, soon removing to the even more fashionable medical area of Harley Street. There he had elegant and beautifully appointed waiting rooms, treatment rooms with his own patent inhalation machine looking for all the world like an upright piano with pipes, and special rooms for use by servants of the patients. He certainly seemed to enjoy a great measure of success, though there were some who whispered that he was careful never to treat anyone who actually was suffering from the disease. It was easy, they said, to produce an inflamed area merely by hard rubbing, and to claim a cure by rubbing less vigorously.

As may be imagined, the medical profession was after his blood, particularly when he put up his shingle in Harley Street itself, the home of the most expensive and fashionable physicians. Long himself was scathing in his contempt for his medical opponents, and said, "Had I practised in obscurity I should not have excited the envy of the profession. My offence was that I practised among the affluent and shared a proportion of those fees which gild the pill of the licentiate." He was also critical of those general practitioners who made several visits to families who could scarce afford their fees, when one visit should have been enough.

He was proud of the fact that he had no medical qualifications of any kind, and had not purchased his diploma from London or Aberdeen without the necessity of taking an examination, as others had done.

Near catastrophe came to Long in 1830, when he treated an Irish girl, Katherine Cashin, for tuberculosis. Unfortunately she seems to have been allergic to Long's liniment and her body became so inflamed and painful that she refused further treatment. Though she was later attended by no less a personage than Sir James Brodie, physician to the king, she died in a few days in terrible agony.

Long was thereupon arrested and accused of manslaughter. At his trial, though many eminent people spoke in his defense, he was convicted and fined the comparatively small sum of five hundred dollars.

Very shortly afterward another patient died after the treatment, and once again Long found himself in the dock accused of manslaughter. This time the evidence was so contradictory that the jury acquitted him, though many considered him to be a very lucky man indeed. Long was evidently more affected by this acquittal than he had been by his conviction, for he immediately began publishing broadsheets defending his method of treatment. One such broadsheet bore the signatures of eighty-six eminent personages, including those of nine members of the peerage and several well-known clerics.

Long's death in 1832, at the age of thirty-four, came as a shock to all. In his will he valued the secret of his liniment at twenty-five thousand dollars, but his brother, who was the sole beneficiary, failed to find a buyer. For a man who promised long life and health to tubercular patients, his own life was tragically short, for he succumbed to the disease he purported to cure, as is the fate of many a quack. But he was a colorful figure in nineteenth-century medicine, and his death left a gap that was never filled, neither in the annals of quackery nor in the hearts of many a "pale but interesting" young lady.

In America there were few quacks then of Long's caliber. The American public, perhaps because of the diversity of religious cults which characterized it at the time, tended to look more toward faith healing than to bizarre medical cures, and several such healers decorate the contemporary scene.

Phineas Quimby of Maine (1802–1866) experimented with hypnotism from the 1830s as a means of healing, and laid the foundation stone of the cult of Christian Science developed later by Mary Baker Eddy (1821–1910), one of his disciples. The early Mormons claimed to "set bones through the faith of Christ" and, to give additional color to the statement, added that "they come together making the noise like the crushing of an old basket."

Another practitioner of faith-healing was Francis Schlatter, who operated in Denver in the 1890s and claimed to have cured thousands merely by touching them. Like a previous owner of this useful gift, the English King Charles II, Schlatter found that healing by touch became something of a chore, and substituted instead the sending of an object that had touched him—in this case a handkerchief. (King Charles substituted coins.) The United States Government had rather less faith in Schlatter's healing powers than had his patients, and accused him of using the mails to perpetrate a fraud. Little was heard of Schlatter afterward.

All these people were opposed to the standard methods of healing and most were violently antagonistic to the medical profession. One legitimate doctor, however, evolved a curative process of his own which enjoyed a huge vogue in America and Britain at the end of the eighteenth century and the beginning of the nineteenth.

This was Elisha Perkins (1741–1799), whose father was a doctor in Connecticut and who himself qualified as a physician from Yale in 1766. Dr. Perkins invented "Tractoration," a process by which illnesses were cured by stroking the patient's body with a double metallic rod, or "Tractor." For many years Perkins worked as a general practitioner in New England, where he achieved a small degree of fame by being a teetotaler in an area where hard drinking was one of the badges of the medical profession, but did little else to make his name known. In 1796 he suddenly produced his "Metallic Tractors," though he never bothered to explain the rationale of this particular form of treatment, except to suggest that it was in some way connected with the Italian Galvani's experiments in making frogs' legs move by "animal magnetism." At first the Tractors, each about four inches long, were made in a small forge in the doctor's house and were claimed to cure "pains in the head, face, teeth, breast, stomach, back and all other joints." He advertised them in the local press, later adding "paralysis and minor deformities" to the list of afflictions they would cure, and sat back to await results. They were not long coming. To his astonishment orders, and later testimonials, began pouring in from all parts of the country, making even more fantastic claims than he himself had dared.

Perkins, always an astute man of business, increased not only the advertising but also the price, which shot up from ten dollars to twenty-five dollars a pair in six months.

By this time the Connecticut Medical Society was getting worried at what it considered blatant quackery by one of its own members, and in 1797 expelled him from the association. But Perkins forged ahead with bigger and better advertisements ("Half-price to doctors and free to members of the clergy"), and achieved his most spectacular sale when George Washington himself bought a pair.

Soon afterward sales began to sag, and Perkins was forced to think of some other lucrative form of unorthodox treatment. In the event this proved to be a much more conventional product, consisting of an Antiseptic Cure for Yellow Fever, a disease then rife in New York. Early in 1799 Perkins traveled to New York to demonstrate his "cure," but within a month he died—of yellow fever!

Across the Atlantic, however, sales of the Metallic Tractors were just beginning to boom, and Elisha's son, Elisha, Jr., went to England to lead a sales drive. So successful was he that by 1803 the Tractors were in such demand and so highly prized that a Perkins Institute was opened in London by the British Medical Association for the purpose of providing Tractors free for those too poor to buy them. This proved to be Perkins' undoing. It is a basic principle of the successful quack that he never undersells his own product, for the faith of the public in a medication is in direct proportion to the money it pays for it. Once the Tractors were available free of charge, there were immediate complaints that they did not work. Perkins decided to call it a day, packed his bags, and returned to America, taking with him the twenty-five thousand dollars he had netted during his London campaign.

While the vogue for Tractoration lasted, one or two British

doctors climbed on the bandwagon with Tractors of their own, notably Dr. John Haygarth of Bath, whose Tractors were made of wood painted to look like metal. According to reports they were just as effective as the genuine Perkins models. In the nearby city of Bristol a surgeon at the local infirmary also augmented his income by making Tractors out of four-inch nails and coating them with sealing wax. Both doctors, despite the ethics of their profession, made a good deal of money in the process.

Perkins was ahead of his time, but by the middle of the nineteenth century the medical quack, so long a feature of the European scene, was well established in America. Here the quackery was less personal, and manifested itself mainly in the proliferation of countless "patent" medicines guaranteed to cure every illness. Some of them had a fair amount of alcohol, as witness Lydia Pinkham's Vegetable Compound, but there was one illness which demanded the most intimate and personal attention.

This was venereal disease, and there were many physicians on both sides of the Atlantic ready to make a quick killing by purporting to have a cure. In America there was a mushrooming of the pernicious "medical institutes" and museums to which guillible but guilty young men were drawn like flies into a honey pot. Once inside they were faced with a dramatic and sickening waxworks exhibition apparently portraying the ravages of VD, and they were quickly convinced that they were showing the early symptoms of the disease. This advice, of course, was "free." The catch came when they committed themselves to the "cure" and found themselves relieved of several hundred dollars.

The scandal of the institutes finally came to a head with the case of the Drs. Kennedy who ran an institute in Detroit. After they told a young and impoverished immigrant, who was getting married, that he had contracted syphilis, the wretched youth went home and shot himself. The autopsy showed quite clearly that he was suffering from no disease of any kind, the result being that the medical brothers hurriedly shut up shop and tried to flee the country. One succeeded, but the other was apprehended and spent the next six months in the penitentiary. All over America such places hurriedly closed down, and the scandal of the quack VD Institute was over.

An equally popular but more legitimate medical racket was the so-called cure for alcoholism. Though there were many patent medicines available for this (mostly consisting of diluted sherry), the main practitioner in this field was Dr. Leslie Keeley of Dwight, Illinois, a man who had once been chief railroad surgeon on the Chicago & Alton.

At Dwight he established his famous sanatorium for alcoholics, based on his "discovery" that gold bichloride reduced the craving for alcohol. As a result of his advertising, drunks by the hundred were soon falling off the trains arriving in Dwight into the arms of Keeley attendants waiting on the platforms. Pausing only for the patient to sign the all-important contract, nurses began treatment immediately with a shot of gold bichloride in the arm. Once inside the clinic gold bichloride was rarely used, and instead a gradual weaning away of the patient from alcohol was substituted, often with satisfactory, if temporary, results. Keeley himself claimed a success rate of 90 percent, but it is doubtful if that figure was ever achieved in terms of permanent cure. Because of his much-publicized use of the highly expensive gold bichloride, Keeley was able to keep his fees extremely high, yet was never short of patients. Over the years he went on to establish some forty institutes in various states in America. There was even talk of establishing a chain in Britain, but the British Medical Association was not impressed and took its stand on an extremely adverse report on the Dwight Institute rendered by Dr. Usher, an Australian doctor who had visited it.

Dr. Keeley died a very rich man in 1900, and the institute still exists today, still under his name but under new management. But now there is no mention of gold bichloride in the treatment, which relies on the modern psychiatric approach, together with the use of certain revulsion therapy drugs. The previous tiny hamlet of Dwight is now a flourishing township, and the old institute buildings are a hospital for veterans.

Keeley's activities demonstrate yet again the very thin borderline existing between quackery and conventional therapy, for at least part of his treatment was in accordance with modern thought on the subject. This is a consideration that must always be borne in mind when considering quack remedies, for not only does faith play a large part in any cure, but modern research is constantly demonstrating that what was once thought to be useless folk medicine had within it a sound scientific idea. It is very apposite to remember that what may be the quack medicine of today may well be the medical milestone of tomorrow.

IX

The International Scene in the Seventeenth and Eighteenth Centuries

THE RAPID RISE and pernicious influence of the quack doctor during the seventeenth and eighteenth centuries was largely due to the way medicine was organized during this period. Doctors attended to the needs of the wealthy, who were in a position to pay, even if they often did so with reluctance, and very occasionally a doctor would treat a destitute person free of charge. But the great mass of the working population in Europe had no access to general physicians, except in circumstances of great urgency, for they could not afford their fees. Instead they had recourse to the quacks, to the itinerant medicine sellers and fairground hucksters, or to the herbalists and apothecaries. And even the apothecaries had to be treated with a certain amount of caution.

By the act of Henry VIII the apothecaries and surgeons had been separated and each given their own guild, though the apothecaries were barred from accepting payment for diagnosis or treatment. Instead, they were allowed to charge for the drugs and medication supplied, something which could, in the event, become as costly as calling in a good physician. A doctor could easily give advice at little cost to himself, but the apothecary, who had to buy his own medicines and dressings wholesale, could not be expected to give them away for nothing.

Both apothecaries and doctors were concerned with this situation, but in England little was done to remedy this state of affairs until the events surrounding the plague of London brought things to a head.

It was in June 1665 that the plague first manifested itself in the rat-infested timber hovels and warehouses near the Thames. For this reason it is often called "The Poore's Plague," though by the time it ended all classes had been affected. The plague was, in reality, a particularly bad outbreak of an epidemic which had never actually died out in England since the Black Death three centuries before. Over the years there had been sporadic outbreaks in ports and riverside towns where the rats, with their cargo of infected fleas, had kept the pestilence alive.

In London that year, as whole families died, their houses were shut and the corpses left for the women called "searchers" to complete their gruesome task of examining the bodies for the telltale mark or "token" that signaled death from plague, before the bodies were heaped into communal burying pits. As the deaths increased, the wealthy fled from the city into the surrounding countryside, and many physicians were among them, either to escape the plague or to keep in contact with their more wealthy patients. The houses of the sick were marked with a cross, and the legend "Lord Have Mercy on Us" put on the door, for there was little to be done by the few doctors remaining in London. At the height of the epidemic whole streets were treated in this manner, and in September 1665 no less than 12,000 people were said to have died in London in one week alone.

Those who took refuge in the countryside to escape the plague, like the poet John Milton, found themselves highly unpopular with the inhabitants of the villages to which they went, for the villagers feared contamination. That their fears were often justified is shown by the fact that by the following year 2500 people had died in the city of Norwich, and in Eyam, a little village in Derbyshire, five out of six of the whole population succumbed when a box of flea-infested clothing was sent to the village from London.

Of those who recorded the progress of the plague, the diarist Samuel Pepys gives many a graphic eyewitness account of life in London during those fateful months. His version is more accurate, if occasionally less dramatic, than is Daniel Defoe's *Journal of the Plague Year*, for the author was only six years old in 1665 and must have obtained much of his material at second-hand.

One of the few physicians who stayed in London during the plague was Dr. Nathaniel Hodges who left the best account of it in his *Loimogia* of 1672 (the Greek word for pestilence is "loimos").

He describes how he rose very early each morning, took a dose of "anti-plague electuary," and then began his rounds, visiting the sick in their own homes. Back home to breakfast and another dose of medicine, and then off once more. At the door of each house strips of wood were burned as a fumigant, and as an additional precaution Dr. Hodges sucked lozenges of myrrh, cinnamon, and angelica root. Each day he worked on until nine or ten o'clock in the evening, when he returned home for his supper, always being careful to take a glass of sack before and after the meal. This, he considered, was the most important safeguard of all, and although on two occasions he experienced the early symptoms of the plague, two glasses of sack on each occasion halted its onset.

He treated his patients by attempting to "sweat" the disease out of them by the use of marigold and other herbs, by insisting on light diet, and by trying to ensure a good supply of fresh air —something which was almost impossible in the stinking hovels in which the disease flourished. Great store was also placed on fumigation with wood rich in resin. Few of these remedies were effective, and during that hot summer of 1665 the carts rumbled the streets of London with their dreadful cry, "Bring out your dead."

By the end of the year the pestilence had begun to abate, and the rich, together with their medical advisers, returned to the capital. Many physicians were troubled in their conscience at the realization of how many poor people had perished, and how few doctors had remained to give them comfort, if little else. Fresh thought was given to a means of providing regular medical attention in London for the needy, and in 1675 a scheme was evolved to provide a dispensary for the poor. Under this scheme the impoverished person could go to the dispensary, where the doctors would give their services free and the apothecaries provide medicines and dressings, if not free, "at the most reasonable rate." The reason why the scheme failed was because the apothecaries, who had to buy their drugs and relied on the profit for their living, could not supply them at low prices without lowering their own income. Many physicians were also opposed to giving their services free, and a violent argument arose between dispensarians and antidispensarians and the scheme came to nothing.

A few years later the apothecaries themselves came forward with an ingenious idea for a dispensary. They undertook to provide medication and dressings free on the understanding that they alone would diagnose the illnesses and provide treatment. This, of course, was not only out of the question but illegal, for the law provided that only a member of the Royal College of Physicians could diagnose and treat disease.

Finally a scheme came into being which excluded the apothecaries completely. In 1698 a dispensary was opened by the Royal College of Physicians itself, where free treatment was given by doctors who bought their own medicaments from the drug wholesalers and supplied them at cost price or even for nothing. The controversy was enshrined in print by a member of the R.C.P., Sir Samuel Garth who, in 1699, published a long, mock-heroic poem on the subject, entitled *The Dispensary*.

The efforts of certain doctors to alleviate the sufferings of the poor by supplying free medical aid did little to raise the status of the profession in the eyes of the nobility. Though the rich families made use of physicians, in many instances they considered them "low" people. In 1661 the daughter of Sir Justinian Isham was courted by the son of Oliver Cromwell's former doctor. She angrily repudiated him, describing him as "a vulgar creature and a sniffling Puritan." In this she was upheld by her father who maintained that "the gentry must make a bulwarke against the Sea of Democracy which was over-running them."

Too often the gentry and nobility expressed their superiority over the medical profession by the simple expedient of forgetting to pay them, making it necessary for doctors to charge inordinate amounts to those honest enough to pay their bills. In 1680, as an example, one London physician was charging $100 for attendance at a confinement, a sum equivalent to about $1500 today. Small wonder that the most fashionable doctors earned amounts far higher than was normal in most other professions, and which were exceeded only by the fees of the most successful quacks. Dr. Richard Mead, a favorite London physician of the time, had an annual income which would represent $150,000 today. But salaries like this were rare outside the capital. Most seventeenth-century doctors were forced to work very long hours to scratch a meager living and frequently had to embark on various kinds of quackery to satisfy their patients and to augment their income.

While this situation existed among doctors in general practice, there were many others who were experimenting and researching at the various hospitals throughout the kingdom.

One of the greatest of these was William Harvey (1578–1657) who qualified at the University of Padua, in Italy, in 1601. Returning to London he was appointed physician in charge at St. Bartholomew's Hospital in London, where he later became lecturer in anatomy and surgery. He held this appointment for the next forty years, during which time he formulated his important theories and findings regarding the circulation of the blood. He was also the author of the first textbook on midwifery to be written by a British doctor.

Harvey, like all innovators and experimenters, had many opponents, most of whom he ignored. An exception was the comments of his great friend Jean Riolan, professor of anatomy in Paris. But Harvey's theories were proved correct by an Italian, Marcello Malpighi (1628–1694), who first used a primitive microscope to observe the flow of blood in the arterial and venous systems.

Much medical research in the seventeenth century was conducted by men who were scientists and physicists, rather than doctors, and among them the name of Robert Boyle (1627–1691) must have pride of place. Boyle proved that life could not be supported without an adequate supply of air, which he showed to be a substance which could be weighed and measured. His friend and colleague, the Cornish scientist Richard Lower (1631–1691), was the first to achieve the successful transfusion of blood from one living animal to another, so leading to experiments on human beings. These, however, proved unsuccessful and frequently fatal, and medicine had to wait until the discovery and classification of blood groups by Karl Landsteiner and Jansky in 1907 before further progress could be made.

In the field of pure medicine, as distinct from surgery or physiology, Dr. Thomas Sydenham (1624–1689) and his teachings took the general practitioner away from academic theories and textbooks and encouraged him to look closely at the patient and to study the symptoms. His brief and concise book *Medical Observations* and his *Treatise on Gout* are models of clarity in describing symptoms and are as accurate today as they were then. Sydenham was a pioneer in the use of iron for anemia, and of the newly discovered cinchona bark for ague and malaria.

A pupil of Sydenham was the rumbustious Dr. Thomas Dover (1660–1742), part pirate and part ship's doctor, who took part in the rescue of Alexander Selkirk (the original Robinson Crusoe) and whose famous powders are still occasionally prescribed today.

Further important contributions to medical knowledge were made in England by Dr. Thomas Willis (1621–1675), who was the first physician to research the structure of the brain, and Francis Glisson (1597–1677), whose work resulted in the correct account of the function of the liver.

On the continent of Europe medical research was also continuing apace. At the famous University of Leyden, in Holland, under Hermann Boerhaave (1668–1738), progress was made in the study of anatomy which had earlier been commemorated in the picture "The Anatomy Lesson" by Rembrandt in 1632. In Germany Friedrich Hoffmann (1660–1742) was studying the effect of various chemicals and drugs on disease and at the same time was taking the opportunity of making a considerable sum on the side by selling his own patent medicines or tonics. In France a notable step forward came in the dissemination of medical knowledge when Nicholas de Blegny, "the royal wound-doctor," published the first medical journal not written in Latin, in 1679. The French Académie des Sciences, founded in 1666 by Louis XIV, also helped to raise the status of the physician, particularly those employed in the armed services.

In Russia the first glimmerings of medical progress had been seen in 1550 when one or two primitive hospitals were established under the supervision of foreign physicians. The status of the Russian doctor was greatly raised under Czar Michael (reigned 1613–1645), who made all doctors members of the nobility and granted them large estates, a proceeding which created untold jealousy.

Russia had its own Plague Year in 1654, the result being the establishment of the country's first medical school four years later. In 1694 Peter Postnikov was the first Russian to graduate as a doctor of medicine in Europe. Under Peter the Great (1672–1725) medicine was completely reorganized and many European doctors were invited to Moscow to teach and to study. Further progress was made by the founding of Russia's first university at Moscow in 1775.

In the two hundred years that have passed since, medical research in Russia has caught up with that in the rest of Europe, and in 1904 the fourth Nobel Prize was awarded to a Russian, Ivan P. Pavlov, for his work on the digestive system.

Not only Russia benefited from the many foreign doctors who went there to teach and study. Most countries of Europe, during this period, saw an exchange of men and ideas which helped to propagate medical knowledge. The University of Leyden was attracting students from far afield, and by the eighteenth century had taken on the ancient mantle of medicine formerly worn by Montpellier in France and Salerno in Italy.

Ties with Europe had always been stronger in Scotland than in England, and it was therefore no coincidence that the first three professors of medicine at the Royal College of Physicians in Edinburgh should have all been trained at Leyden. Among them was Archibald Pitcairne (1652–1713) who had also studied in Paris, and who had taken holy orders and qualified as a lawyer before turning to medicine. He lived to become Scotland's most famous physician, and was an ardent supporter of Harvey's theories regarding the circulation of the blood at a time when such ideas were not universally popular. Toward the end of his life he was invited back to Leyden as professor of medicine, but after a year was forced to resign and return to Edinburgh for family reasons. When he died, his will provided that a jeroboam of wine should be purchased and kept to be drunk when the Stuarts eventually returned to the throne, an event which he apparently assumed to be imminent. History was to decide otherwise. In 1800 a trio of medical men in Edinburgh decided to restore Pitcairne's tomb, by then falling into neglect, and celebrated the occasion by disposing of the jeroboam of wine.

One of Pitcairne's students of Leyden was John Monro, who was responsible for the establishment of the medical school of Edinburgh, and one of Monro's sons went on to become a brilliant teacher of anatomy. There is a story that while the son was waiting for the corpse of a recently hanged female to be brought in for dissection, the "body" suddenly revived and sat up, much to the embarrassment of the assembled company, including Monro. The girl who narrowly escaped death to suffer this humiliating public exposure lived on for many years, and became known in the district as "Half-hanged Maggie Dickson."

Scottish-born doctors have made very many notable contributions to medical knowledge, and in the seventeenth and eighteenth centuries the medical schools of Glasgow and Edinburgh were equal to any found in Europe.

In the field of obstetrics a notable figure was Dr. William Smellie (1697–1763), who was Scottish-born and studied at Glasgow. He soon moved to London where his lectures on midwifery made him famous, and his *Treatise on Midwifery* (1752) cleared up much of the superstition and incorrect information surrounding the subject. He was also the first to use publicly the obstetric forceps invented about 1600 by Peter Chamberlen, a Huguenot refugee, but kept a trade secret by his family for seven generations. Another Scot was William Hunter (1718–1783), who also practiced obstetrics in London and took over from Smellie on his death.

But it was his brother, John Hunter (1728–1793), who is better remembered as a surgeon, lecturer, and avid collector of any out-of-the-way object or information that could further medical knowledge. In London he became a fashionable physician, with a large house in Leicester Square which contained his living quarters, his office, a lecture theater, and a museum. One of his most famous pupils was the extraordinarily named American, Philip Syng Physick (1768–1837), who was later to become professor of surgery at Pennsylvania Hospital.

The medical scene in eighteenth-century Europe is also remarkable for the number of medically qualified men whose fame rests not on medicine, but on their achievements in the arts or politics. In England, Tobias Smollett (1721–1771) became famous as the author of *The Adventures of Roderick Random,* and the poet and playwright Oliver Goldsmith (1728–1774) had qualified as a doctor in 1754. The poet John Keats (1795–1821) was also a doctor, as was the East Anglian poet George Crabbe (1754–1832).

In France two medical figures have put their permanent mark on history by their association with the French Revolution. One was Dr. Joseph Guillotin (1738–1814) who invented the guillotine, the other, the political activist Jean Marat (1743–1793) murdered in his bath by Charlotte Corday. In Germany medicine has given us the poet Johann Schiller (1759–1805).

In England a man who achieved some fame as a minor poet, but who was also responsible for one of the most important steps forward in medicine, was Edward Jenner (1749–1823). He was an ordinary country doctor, though a pupil of John Hunter, who preferred the quiet rural round of daily life in Berkeley, Gloucestershire, to seeking fame and fortune in London. His fame rests on his experiments in inoculating farm laborers with the exudation from cowpox sores as a method of avoiding them contracting the far more virulent and deadly smallpox, the scourge of England for many centuries. A quiet and self-effacing man, Jenner desired no glory for himself, but modestly made his findings known in a medical journal. The result was an immediate drop in the incidence and morbidity of smallpox, and a paving of the way for the later techniques of vaccination and immunology.

While it was customary in the eighteenth century for British medical students to go to the continent of Europe for the purpose of study and graduation, American medical students crossed the Atlantic to Edinburgh for this purpose. Among the many who did so one of the most important was John Morgan (1735–1789) who qualified in Edinburgh and returned home to found that cradle of American medical knowledge, the University of Pennsylvania Medical College in 1765. On the outbreak of the

War of Independence he was made director-general of the army medical department, but owing to his unorthodox political views was dismissed and replaced by William Shippen, who was also an Edinburgh graduate. At Philadelphia, Morgan was followed later by yet another graduate from Edinburgh, Benjamin Rush (1745–1813). Rush was also a formidable political figure, an author, and signer of the Declaration of Independence. He was treasurer of the U.S. Mint, and established the first free dispensary for the poor in America in 1796.

On the edge of the medical scene in London during most of the eighteenth century was the vast and uncouth figure of Dr. Samuel Johnson, often described as the only man who talked his way into history. Johnson (1709–1784) was a doctor of literature, not of medicine, but his insatiable curiosity caused him to follow the byways of medicine and all matters scientific. He wrote biographies of many medical men, including Thomas Sydenham and Boerhaave, and in 1743 contributed several pages to Dr. Robert James's gargantuan *Medical Dictionary*. Being a sick man all his life, he was constantly in need of medical attention himself, and was attended by many doctors, most of whom were put off by his surly manner and unwillingness to cooperate. He did not endear himself to them, either, by his habit of consulting other doctors by post while his own doctors were treating him at his bedside. One of his doctors was the equally eccentric Dr. Richard Brocklesby (1722–1797) who bequeathed in his will two thousand dollars to Edmund Burke, and then gave it to him in his lifetime because he thought he needed the money. He also offered an annuity to Johnson to go and live in a warmer climate, which the irascible writer refused on the grounds that he was "accelerating towards death." He lived another thirty years!

Dr. Johnson is also one of the final links with that curious custom of the royal touch as a cure for scrofula. As a child, Johnson had been brought from Lichfield to London to be "touched" by Queen Anne, the last British monarch to indulge in this custom. No cure had been effected, and Johnson remained a sufferer the whole of his life.

On the other side of Europe, in Austria, another cure by means of touch was being developed at this time by Dr. Franz Mesmer (1734–1815) and was based on his theory of "animal magnetism." This he believed to be an invisible fluid which, when discharged from the operator to the patient, could cure disease. Like many other prophets before and since he was derided in his own country and decided to journey elsewhere. He chose Paris, and there he had better luck and impressed many doctors with his own rather unusual form of treatment. For this a tub was required, and iron filings and broken glass were put in and covered with water. Rods protruded from the lid, and when patients gripped these rods the magnetism flowed through them, so alleviating their symptoms. Later Mesmer announced that he could transfer magnetism from himself to his patients without bodily contact and by merely gazing at them until they went into a trance. When they came out of the trance, all symptoms had vanished and would not return.

This became known as "mesmerism" or "hypnotism," and though it lapsed after Mesmer's death in 1815, it was revived in late-Victorian times and is once again undergoing a fresh assessment as the forerunner of the modern technique of psychotherapy.

The eighteenth century was an age of realism. It was a time of invention rather than of theory, as the Industrial Revolution got under way. It was also a slightly self-satisfied age, and the various diagnostic aids to medicine which were invented were looked upon largely as the final seal of perfection on treatments which were unlikely to be bettered.

In 1707 Sir John Floyer, a physician of Lichfield, introduced his "Physician's Pulse Watch" which differed from normal chronometers of the time by having a second hand. During the course of the century the clinical thermometer gradually came into common use, and in Vienna Leopold Augenbrucker, noting that the cellerman in his father's tavern gauged the contents of the wine barrels by tapping them, adapted that procedure in assessing the amount of fluid on the chest of sufferers from bronchitis. At the turn of the century the Frenchman, René Théophile Hyacinthe Laënnec (1781–1826), had invented the stethoscope after seeing children playing with rolled tubes of paper to magnify the sound.

Another innovator who flourished at the end of the eighteenth century was the German doctor Samuel Hahnemann (1755–1843) the founder of homeopathy. For many years the cure of disease by herbs and drugs had been carried out on the principle that "the more you give the better it will work." The result was the habit of prescribing huge quantities of drugs as a dose, or to include in a mixture as many as twenty different ingredients. There had already been some opposition to this practice, and the famous preacher John Wesley had thundered against doctors and apothecaries in his *Primitive Physick* published in 1747.

John Wesley would certainly have approved of Hahnemann's homeopathy, for it was based on principles diametrically opposed to the taking of large or complex dosages. The idea was really an updating of the ancient doctrine of signatures but applied only to symptoms and not to external appearance. Belladonna, for example, when taken in tiny doses, produced symptoms similar to scarlet fever: it could therefore be taken to cure this disease. Again, ipecacuanha seemed to precipitate a mild form of asthma: it was therefore the right drug to use in the treatment of this complaint.

Hahnemann also stipulated that only one form of medication should be taken at one time. But it is his third proviso that has remained firmly fixed in the public mind—that infinitesimally small doses of the chosen drug are all that is needed to effect a cure, and that the original mother tincture can be diluted very many times and still retain its action. Needless to say, in propounding this theory Hahnemann had his critics, the most vocal being the apothecaries, who saw the sale of herbs and drugs being ruinously reduced if the idea caught on. In many countries, doctors, too, scoffed at the idea, but by no means all. In France the president of the Assembly refused to take any action against those who practiced the new art of homeopathy, maintaining that if it did not do what was claimed for it, it would die a natural death, but if it really worked, then it was an important step forward in treatment. In England a forward-looking general practitioner, Harvey Quin, took the trouble to go to Germany and learn the theory of homeopathy thoroughly, returning to London to become Britain's first homeopathic doctor. Yet despite this, and despite the fact that the British royal family were enthusiastic homeopaths, homeopathy today has a far lower standing in England than it has in America, France, or Germany.

X

The Doctor Goes West

THE FIRST PART of the seventeenth century was an era of exploration and discovery, not only geographically but also in the sciences. Men like Harvey and Sydenham were beginning to question the ancient authorities of Galen and Hippocrates at the same time as the first permanent settlers in the New World began to probe their way inland.

It was unfortunate, if not downright tragic, that in America exploration of the new continent came first, while the old ideas of the four humors still maintained in medicine, and treatment was still largely a matter of witchcraft and superstition.

The early colonists in the New World experienced hardships such as never existed in England. It was in April 1607 that the first contingent sighted the twin capes of Chesapeake Bay and landed in Virginia after a sea voyage of ninety-six days. It had been a grueling experience. Huddled into three tiny ships, with accommodation severely limited, food and provisions sparse, and an almost total lack of hygiene, many had not survived the journey.

Perhaps they were the fortunate ones, for those who landed were to endure for many months hardships that have been described as the most tragic of any group of settlers.

Not that the settlers came entirely unprepared. The London Company, which had organized the venture, had earlier surveyed the coastline and had even penetrated a few miles inland before returning home. They had expected that disease would take its toll and had warned the settlers accordingly. It is likely that if these warnings and instructions had been heeded, much hardship and loss of life would have been avoided. As it was, those who disembarked were more concerned with protecting themselves from marauding Indians rather than with the avoidance of disease, and their actions were geared to this from the start. Firstly they required a site where they could have good visibility up and down the river and also survey the hills from where the enemy was likely to come. Accordingly they established themselves at a site some thirty miles upstream, at a place later called Jamestown, in low-lying and marshy land bordering the brackish waters of the estuary.

For men already debilitated by disease and the rigors of the Atlantic crossing, building an encampment and hunting for food in these conditions were herculean tasks. One by one they succumbed to dietary disorders and unfamiliar disease, until by the autumn of 1607 only forty remained out of the hundred who had landed.

George Percy, one of the first arrivals in Jamestown, graphically described the terrible conditions which prevailed.

> Our men are destroyed with cruel disease, as swellings, fluxes, burning fevers, and by wars, and some departed suddenly. But for the most part they died of famine. There were never Englishmen left in a foreign country in such misery as we were, in this newly-discovered Virginia. We watched every three nights, lying on the bare cold ground, what weather soever came; working all the next day, which brought our men to be most feeble wretches. Our food was but a small can of barley sod in water to five men a day: our drink cold water taken out of the river, which was at flood very salty, at low tide full of slime and filth. Our men groaned day and night in every corner of the fort most pitiful to hear. If there were any conscience in men it would make their hearts bleed to hear the the pitiful murmurings and outcries of our sick men, without relief every night and day for the space of six weeks; some departed out of this world, many times three or four in a night, in the morning their bodies trailed out of their cabins like dogs to be buried.

Between 1607 and 1621 it is estimated that more than four thousand settlers landed on the shores of America, yet in 1624 the entire white population (including babies born since landing) numbered less than two thousand.

Medical attention for the colonists was sparse, for no qualified doctors were found among the first settlers. Admittedly, there were a few with a smattering of medical knowledge, such as "Doctor" Samuel Fuller, who landed with the *Mayflower* and whose wife became the first midwife of the colony. Others were medical students who made the journey for experience, but soon returned home to complete their studies. The first qualified physician to make his permanent home in the New World was Dr. John Pott, who arrived in 1625 and was later to be appointed governor of Virginia in 1628.

Those like Pott who were concerned with sickness and matters of health in the New World brought with them the old ideas of Galen and the four humors—ideas which were soon to become outmoded by the theories of Sydenham and Harvey. In their contact with the Indians the settlers found themselves face to face with the beliefs of primitive man.

With the Indians the medicine man or witch doctor still played an important part. Cures were effected by ritual, magic, and sacrifice. John Lawson, surveyor-general to the colonists in North Carolina, gives a vivid description of the manner in which the medicine men of the Seneca tribe treated their patients:

> As soon as the doctor comes into the cabin, the sick person is set on a mat or skin, stark-naked. In this manner the patient lies when the conjurer appears, and the King of that nation comes to attend him with a rattle made of a gourd with peas in it. Then the doctor begins and utters some words very softly; afterwards he smells the patient's navel and belly and sometimes scarifies him a little with a flint, or an instrument made of rattlesnake teeth for this purpose: then he sucks the patient and gets out a mouthful of blood and serum which he spits into a bowl of water. Then he begins to mutter and talk apace, and at last cuts capers till he gets into a sweat, so that a stranger would think him running mad, and now and then sucking the patient. At last you will see the doctor all over dropping sweat, and scarcely able to utter one word, having quite spent himself: and then he will cease for a while, and so begin again till he comes in the same pitch of raving and seeming madness as before; all this time the sick person never so much as moves, although doubtless the sucking and the

lancing must be a great punishment to them. At last the conjurer makes an end, and tells the patient's friends whether the patient will live or die; and then one that waits at this ceremony takes the blood away and buries it in the ground at a place unknown to anyone but he that inters it.

Unfortunately for the colonists and for the Indians, sickness and disease seem to have increased rapidly in both communities once the settlers had arrived. The newcomers were suffering from fevers and dysentery caused by the heat and the unaccustomed surroundings, while the Indians soon began to show symptoms of an epidemic disease they had picked up from the colonists.

There are many theories as to what exactly this disease was, ranging from bubonic plague to yellow fever, though later research has discounted both of these. It is possible that the disease was measles, a complaint which, though common in Europe, was long-standing enough to have conferred some degree of immunity in the population and which affected children far more than adults. But the American Indians had never had experience of it, and had therefore no built-in resistance to it, the result being an epidemic of vast and virulent proportions which decimated whole tribes.

According to a contemporary account by John Josselyn, the Indian method of dealing with the contagion was to put the patient in a wigwam and cover it with bark "so close that no air can enter into it." A fire was lit near the patient until he was sweating profusely and was seen to be semiconscious, at which point he was quickly removed from the wigwam and thrown bodily into the nearest river or lake. Says Josselyn laconically, "They either recover or give up the Ghost."

In most instances the settlers adopted the less spectacular methods of healing practiced by the Indians, such as recourse to herbs and the favorite treatment of short periods of starvation. Very occasionally they were able to demonstrate the superiority of European methods of healing, but, if they did so, enlisted the certain enmity of the medicine man, who felt his position being weakened.

A happy example of the white man's success in healing oc-curred in the early days of the Plymouth Colony, when Massasoit, chief of the Wampanoag Indians, fell ill in 1621 and the medicine men were able to hold out no hope. Massasoit had always been friendly to the colonists, and when news of his illness was received, two settlers, Edward Winslow, a *Mayflower* colonist and later governor of Plymouth Colony, and John Hamden made a special visit to him. Winslow, in his famous *Good News from New England* (1624), described how Massasoit was cured by Winslow and Hamden carefully scraping his tongue and mouth so that he could swallow, and then feeding him with chicken broth. The elders of the tribe were so impressed by this feat (Massasoit was to live another forty years) that they insisted that Winslow should scrape the tongue of every male member of the tribe, a duty which he carried out with some reluctance, as he says, "though it were much offensive to me, not being accustomed to such poisonous savours."

There is little doubt that Winslow's action in this matter saved the lives of many settlers, for so grateful were the chiefs that they revealed the existence of a plot by another tribe to murder the colonists, and Massasoit was to remain their trusted ally and friend to the end of his life.

A qualified physician who exerted much influence among the colonists was Dr. John Winthrop (1606–1676), who was not only a doctor, but also a barrister and an early member of the Royal Society of Arts in England. He it was who encouraged the Indian custom of fast days among the colonists to combat such diseases as influenza, diphtheria, and whooping cough which had followed them to the New World.

Smallpox also ravaged the colony from 1663, and occasioned the writing of the first medical tract to be printed in America. It was written by a Boston doctor named Thomas Thacher, and bore the somewhat unwieldy title: *Brief Rule to guide the common people of New-England how to order themselves and theirs in the Small Pocks and the Measels.*

By the beginning of the eighteenth century, doctors and physicians were beginning to be found in most communities of any size. Some had come direct from Europe, others had been born in the New World and had returned to Europe to qualify, mainly at Leyden or at Edinburgh. Oliver Wendell Holmes

(1808–1894), himself a physician, has described the typical doctor of those early days:

> His pharmacopeia consisted mainly of simples. . . . St. John's Wort, Clownes All-Heale, with Spurge and Fennel, Saffron and Parsely, Elder and Snakeroot, with opium in some form, and roasted rhubarb and the Four Great Cold Seeds, and the two resins . . . with the more familiar Scammony and Jalap and Black Hellebore. He would order Iron now and then and possibly an occasional dose of Antimony. He would perhaps have had a rheumatic patient wrapped in the skin of a wolf or wild cat, and in case of a malignant fever with 'purples' or of an obstinate King's Evil he might have prescribed a certain black powder, which had been made by calcining toads in an earthern pot. Sydenham had not yet cleansed the Pharmacopeia of its perilous stuff, but there is no doubt that the more sensible doctors of the day knew well enough that a good honest herb-tea which amused the patient and his nurse was all that was required to carry him through all common disorders.

Medicine in eighteenth-century America was dominated by the great inoculation controversy. Oddly enough this was precipitated by two well-known men, Cotton Mather and Benjamin Franklin, neither of whom were doctors.

It began when Cotton Mather (1663–1728), the Boston preacher and writer, was elected to membership in the Royal Society of London in 1713. As a member he received the *Transactions* of the society, and there read an account of how people in Turkey were cured of the smallpox by having a small amount of pus from a smallpox victim put into a scratch on the skin. The person so treated had only a very minor outbreak, which left no disfiguring marks, and was made immune for life from further attacks.

At that time smallpox was a scourge in New England, and the fatality rate was distressingly high. Cotton Mather recognized this procedure as being a useful means of reducing the incidence of the disease, but, though reasonably knowledgeable on matters medical, was not in a position to undertake this technique himself.

Accordingly he sought assistance from a well-known Boston doctor, Zabdiel Boylston (1679–1766), who in 1721 first experimented with inoculation on his own son of thirteen, and on two black servants. Dr. Boylston later exposed them to the disease by taking them to the local pesthouse, but none of the three contracted the pox.

Spurred on by this success, Boylston undertook a mass inoculation of his patients when a severe epidemic swept Boston the following year. Unfortunately the death rate was comparatively high, even among those he had inoculated. In addition it became known that those who had been inoculated, while themselves immunized against the disease, could still pass it on to other people. Local feeling, led by the other physicians of Boston, turned against Cotton Mather and Dr. Boylston, who were accused of spreading the disease. Boylston's house was set on fire and he was attacked in the street, while a bomb was thrown through Mather's window. Leading the opposition to inoculation were the brothers James and Benjamin Franklin, who denounced it in their newspaper the *New England Courant*. The Massachusetts House of Representatives passed a bill making inoculation illegal, but before it became law, the tide suddenly turned the other way. Fresh outbreaks of smallpox were found to be much reduced, and suddenly the value of inoculation was appreciated. Benjamin Franklin himself, another amateur of medicine, was later to say how bitterly he regretted not having his four-year-old son inoculated, for the child died of smallpox.

Though the practice gradually spread throughout America, it was not universally accepted, and in 1747 Governor George Clinton of New York issued a proclamation banning it. In other areas the danger of inoculated people spreading the disease was partly overcome by the establishment of "inoculation farms" where "Ladies and Gentlemen, who wish to have the smallpox by this safe and easy method, may be boarded and have faithful attendance on them."

It was Benjamin Franklin (1706–1790) who was responsible for establishing the first hospital in America, on the suggestion of his friend Dr. Thomas Bond, and in 1752 this was opened in Philadelphia and became the Pennsylvania Hospital. It was also in Philadelphia that the first medical school in America was opened by Dr. John Morgan in 1765. Members of the staff played a large part in the establishment of the medical department of the Continental Army when the Revolution came, though political intrigue and jealousy resulted in the dismissal of the first two chiefs, Drs. Benjamin Charles and John Morgan, for treason.

The war over, American medicine once more began to benefit from the medical research that had been continuing in Europe, and in 1798 Edward Jenner's remarkable treatise on vaccination, as distinct from inoculation, caused a sensation on both sides of the Atlantic. In 1800 a deputation representing American Indian tribes traveled to London to thank him personally and to bring him gifts.

As in Europe, American medicine was now moving out of the era of superstition and folklore and becoming scientific. Country doctors had much easier access, through medical journals, to the research and discoveries being carried on in the hospitals of the big cities. Yet the old ideas took a long time to die. Particularly difficult to eradicate was the idea that all illness and epidemics were a sign of God's anger for transgressions, an attitude that was seen in all its barbarity at the time of the first great cholera epidemic in New York in 1832.

For centuries cholera had been a disease confined entirely to the Orient, but in the early years of the nineteenth century it suddenly began to spread across Europe. It reached England early in 1832, and in America the seaboard towns of Boston, Philadelphia, Baltimore, and New York waited nervously for the epidemic to cross the Atlantic by ship. Few really believed that the ocean would provide an adequate barrier, for transatlantic trade with the cholera-ridden countries of Europe was continuing unabated.

When cholera had first reached France, some American doctors had traveled to Europe to study the disease, and they returned bringing some hope. It was obvious, they said, that cholera was attacking only those "predisposed" to contract it, that is, those living in poverty, filth, and squalor. It attacked the lazy and the godless, who would not shift for themselves, and was therefore unlikely to make much progress in the America of Andrew Jackson whose inhabitants, upright, healthy, and God-fearing, lived in a land particularly blessed by the Almighty.

Even when cholera finally did cross the Atlantic and was reported in Montreal early in June of that year, most American cities, and New York in particular, were certain that an overhaul of the street-cleaning system and household hygiene would be enough to avoid the spread of the disease. Householders were encouraged to clean out their homes and deposit the garbage on the streets, but in New York the scheme was not followed through, the garbage remained uncollected, and the citizens lost interest.

News of the arrival of cholera in Canada had been received with trepidation by the people and there was the beginning of an exodus from the larger towns such as New York, Albany, and Philadelphia into the surrounding countryside. On the twenty-sixth of June 1832 an Irish immigrant dockworker, recently arrived from Montreal, was sent home from work with violent stomach pains. A doctor attended him the next morning, and though his condition had improved overnight, his wife and two children were down with the same symptoms. Within two days the family was dead, and the doctor (together with the colleagues he had consulted) was forced to diagnose Asiatic cholera, the first case in the United States.

A Board of Health was formed in New York, but it seemed singularly reticent about the matter and oddly unwilling to admit that cholera had been diagnosed. The medical profession of the city took exception at this attempted cover-up and formed a special Cholera Committee. On the second of July the committee publicly announced that nine cases of cholera had been diagnosed in the city of New York, of which only one had survived.

The Medical Association and its Cholera Committee were immediately attacked by the New York Board of Health and by various business interests, for scaremongering and creating panic. In particular the prominent banker, John Pintard, accused the Cholera Committee of "impertinent interference" and said it was sabotaging the business life of the city by spreading alarmist rumors.

But, despite Pintard and his business associates, the truth was soon known, and the flood of citizens fleeing the towns that had begun earlier in the year now rose to a torrent. Even the Board of Health in New York was forced to admit that cholera had arrived and was taking its dreadful toll. On the fifth of July the Court of Sessions discharged all paupers from its almshouses, and felons and convicts were removed from prison and transported to the comparative safety of Blackwells Island. The board also requisitioned various abandoned buildings to serve as cholera hospitals, but ran into difficulty in finding staff to man them. Physicians were encouraged to treat victims in their homes, and a reward of twenty dollars was suggested for every doctor who proved he had cured a patient.

From the very beginning the attitude of most thinking folk in the State of New York was that cholera was "the scourge of the sinful." It developed, it was noted, in the areas of the city where the pimps and prostitutes lived, where thieving and drunkenness abounded, and where living conditions were intolerable, due to idleness and sloth. Cholera was obviously a weapon sent by the Lord to punish all such evildoers.

The Western Sunday School Messenger explained the matter to its young and impressionable readers as follows:

> Drunkards and filthy, wicked people of all descriptions are swept away in heaps, as if the Holy God could no longer bear to see their wickedness, just as we sweep away a mass of filth when it has become so corrupt that we cannot bear it. The cholera is not *caused* by intemperance and filth in themselves, but it is a *scourge*, a *rod* in the hand of God . . .

It soon became apparent that this was not only a morally unsound argument, but even worse, a gross oversimplification. It was noted that worthy citizens of substance were being carried off, a phenomenon, in the early days, attributed to the fact that they must have been secret sinners and indulging in vice. This attitude, predictably, was found largely among the clergy, and was believed by millions. It did not, however, find much support among the Roman Catholic clergy, many of whose flock were the alcoholic Irishmen alleged to be the partial cause of the trouble.

It was certainly not the view of the medical profession, who did not approve at all of the Almighty being invoked in the guise of a bringer of disease, though they were very much divided among themselves as to the real cause of the outbreak. Treatment varied enormously, the most common form being the letting of vast quantities of blood from patients, though great faith was placed in massive doses of mercury. The skin was kept warm by rubbing with cayenne pepper, chalk, and calomel (another mercuric compound), and patients were assured that when they began to show unmistakable signs of mercury poisoning, the cholera was leaving them.

Other doctors pinned their faith on tobacco-smoke enemas, electric shock, and saline injections into the veins. As diarrhea was one of the earliest symptoms, it was suggested by the practical-minded Dr. Thomas Spencer of New York that the rectum should be plugged with sealing wax, though this no doubt, may be classified merely as a stop gap solution.

Many physicians had followed their patients into the country, as had happened during the plague of London almost two hundred years earlier, and they had met resistance from villagers who feared that cholera was being spread among them. One doctor was actually murdered for this reason. The result was a shortage of doctors in most towns, a situation that played into the hands of the hordes of quacks who were quick to cash in on the situation. Unqualified practitioners of medicine abounded, in particular the adherents of Samuel Thomson, founder of Thomsonianism, or herbal medicine, in which drugs of nonorganic origin were barred and only "natural" plants or herbs used. Herb mixtures were prepared and patented in do-it-yourself packs and patients encouraged to treat themselves. Thomsonians looked forward to the day when all the learned professions, doctors, barristers, and clergy alike, would be disbanded and "men and women will become their own priests, physicians and lawyers."

Charles E. Rosenberg, in his *The Cholera Years* (1962), quotes from some verses written by Thomson in 1836 which summarize the attitude of the cult toward the professions:

> *The nest of college-birds are three,*
> *Law, Physic and Divinity;*
> *And while these three remain combined,*
> *They keep the world oppressed and blind.*

On Lab'rers money lawyers feast,
Also the Doctor and the Priest.

✸   ✸   ✸   ✸   ✸

The Priest pretends to save the soul,
Doctors to make the body whole;
For money lawyers make their plea,
We'll save it and dismiss the three.

✸   ✸   ✸   ✸   ✸   ✸

Come freemen all, unveil your eyes,
If you this slavish yoke despise;
Now is the time to be set free
From Priests' and Doctors' slavery.

Certainly the medical profession was divided enough in its opinions on the treatment and eradication of cholera to instill little confidence in ordinary people. To most doctors it was caused by a "miasma" or "atmospheric impurity," though it was recognized that this atmosphere was created by filth, garbage, and wretched living conditions. Even the establishment of quarantines by the city authorities was attacked as "flattering vulgar prejudices" and was considered an unwarranted interference by the bureaucracy.

In any event the epidemic died down in the fall of 1832, largely because of an improvement in public hygiene, by attempts to improve the lot of the poor by providing work for the unemployed, and by the free issue of bread and soup to the hungry. In this context, and in the actual treatment of the sick in the hospital and the home, finance played a significant part, for nurses and other workers could not be persuaded to attend the cholera hospitals without high fees. In Lexington, Kentucky, nurses were not available at any fee at all, and visitors and old people were pressed into service. In other hospitals the sick looked after themselves, but in some cities, such as Baltimore, Philadelphia, and Cincinnati, the nuns of the Sisters of Charity undertook the work, and many fell victims themselves.

Temperance workers in all areas rejoiced that cholera was apparently proving the connection between misfortune, illness, and strong drink, despite the fact that in some districts whiskey and gin were both recommended as safeguards against the disease.

By October 1832 the epidemic was officially considered to be over. Minor outbreaks flared up in the spring of 1833 and again in 1834, but soon the cholera hospitals were closed, the boards of health disbanded, and the legal requirements controlling public hygiene largely forgotten. Metropolitan America returned to its pre-1832 complacency—until cholera struck again in 1849.

This time it first flared up in that New York district known as Five Points, having once again been brought by ship from Europe. As before, hygiene in the area, and in much of New York, was virtually nonexistent, the cleaning of the city streets being left to the hordes of hogs that roamed at will disposing of the garbage and, as one scandalized Englishman put it, "almost pushing citizens off the sidewalks." An attempt to remove the hogs, thought to be a contributory factor to the spread of the disease, only made matters worse by leaving the garbage uneaten, and in addition created riots among the poor of the city who depended on the hogs for cheap food.

The epidemic of 1849 traveled quickly across the country, spread by the revolution in transport and by the peregrinations of thousands of forty-niners who took it with them across the continent. Reports received from Belleville, Illinois, Madison, Indiana, and Lavaca, Texas, indicated that fifteen to twenty citizens of each town were dying every day, a rate that continued for several weeks.

As in the 1832 epidemic, treatment consisted mainly of bloodletting, cayenne pepper, and mercury, though this time there was a distinct vogue for sulfur in any form, usually as candles to dispel the "miasma."

In the absence of any positive cure being provided by the doctors, the status of the medical profession in America fell to a new low level, most practitioners being regarded as uneducated quacks. This was not helped by the legislatures in several towns removing all legal restrictions on doctoring, so that anyone could claim to be a physician. This action was carried out in South Carolina and in Maryland in 1838 and in New York State in 1844. In Iowa only six months' "reading" of medical books was required to become a doctor. This situation, coupled with the widespread advertising of patent medicines in the newspapers from the 1840s, encouraged the theories of self-medication expounded by Thomson, though now it did not stop at herbal cures.

It was in this kind of atmosphere that the 1849 epidemic waxed and then gradually abated, though cholera remained active in one town or another in America well into 1854. For the medical profession the outbreaks had been a disaster. Instead of gaining increased prestige by their ability to control the disease, the doctors had found the reverse applied, and the way was left open for homeopathy, hydropathy, herbalism, and various other medical cults all combining to undermine the doctors' standing in the community.

By the beginning of the Civil War things had begun to readjust themselves, and though the gold-headed cane of the eighteenth-century physician was never to be seen again, the profession was once more becoming respectable. As is usual in wartime, conditions speeded up medical research, particularly in the field of surgery.

In hygiene progress had been slow, but in 1854 a London doctor named John Snow (1813–1858) had been investigating an outbreak of cholera in the city, and had proved conclusively that the disease was spread by contaminated water. When cholera once more struck America in 1866, Snow's ideas had been accepted in the Union for more than ten years, and the work of Pasteur in Paris had accustomed doctors to the concept of cholera being caused by a microorganism. The threat of another epidemic in 1866 brought immediate action. Streets were instantly cleared, a panel of health inspectors (all doctors) was formed, and citizens encouraged to report all offenses against the sanitary regulations. The medical boards once more swung into action, and as soon as the first deaths in New York were reported, teams were out disinfecting the belongings and clothing of the victims, with sulfur candles well in evidence for fumigating. Other cities were still not well prepared at first. Chicago had no Board of Health and Cincinnati had no hospital. But these matters were quickly rectified once cholera in New York had been confirmed (though in Cincinnati not until ninety deaths had occurred), and over most of the country the epidemic was contained.

The most important aspect of the 1866 outbreak was the changed attitude of the authorities. No longer was cholera the "scourge of the sinful" and the visitation of God on those who did not conform. As Charles Rosenberg has commented, jeremiads against the immorality of postwar America became everyday newspaper fare, often alongside articles on how best to avoid the plague, but no longer were the two connected.

A changed attitude toward cholera went step by step with new attitudes toward hygiene and the spread of disease. The new graduates from the Philadelphia Medical School were also carrying new ideas to the countryside and doing much to advance medical knowledge generally.

Such a man was Daniel Drake (1785–1852), a peripatetic physician who worked in very many different localities disseminating the most up-to-date medical ideas. He established medical schools at Cincinnati, edited the *Western Journal of the Medical and Physical Sciences,* and wrote an important book based on a thirty-year study of illness and disease in the Mississippi Valley. Though he never visited Europe he was well aware of the latest developments in medicine and became a highly regarded and influential physician. Coming from a family living in the utmost poverty, he has been described as the most picturesque figure in American medicine.

Equally picturesque and certainly as imaginative was his exact contemporary, Dr. William Beaumont (1785–1853). He, too, traveled extensively and was a pioneer in gastric surgery. One of his patients was a Canadian trapper, Alexis St. Martin, who had a large hole in his stomach wall caused by a gunshot wound. Beaumont treated the trapper in such a way that the hole was never totally occluded, and allowed him to examine at any time the working of the gastric system and the action of the digestive juices. Beaumont followed the trapper about for some years in order to pursue his studies, and in 1833 wrote his famous book, *Experiments and Observations on the Gastric Juice and the Physiology of Digestion.*

American medicine has always been to the fore in surgery, and in 1809 a brilliant pioneer in this field, Ephraim McDowell (1771–1830), successfully removed the ovaries of a farmer's wife in the days before antiseptics and anesthetics, so performing the first true ovariotomy. Conditions were primitive, and the patient had to travel sixty miles on horseback for the operation. Three weeks later she was home again and lived another thirty-two years.

An eminent gynecologist of a later generation was James Marion Sims (1813–1883) who became famous both in America and in Europe for the first successful removal of vaginal fistula.

Great progress was also made toward the turn of the century in the control of malaria. The disease had first been investigated by the French army doctor and bacteriologist, Charles Louis Laveran (1845–1922), who studied it in Algeria. In 1897 the Englishman, Sir Ronald Ross (1857–1932) had made a great advance when he demonstrated the association between the spread of malaria and the habit of the *Anopholes* mosquito.

As for yellow fever, it was an American Army surgeon, Major Walter Reed (1851–1902), who, in 1900, in conjunction with James Carroll, Jesse Lazear, and Aristides Agramonte, proved conclusively that the disease was spread by the mosquito known as *Aëdes aegypti*. With this knowledge it was possible virtually to eradicate the disease, a matter of enormous significance in the construction of the Panama Canal under General William Gorgas, from 1904 to 1913.

Of great importance to the American medical scene in the early years of the twentieth century were the Mayo brothers, William James (1861–1939) and Charles Horace (1865–1939). Their father, William Worrall Mayo (1819–1911), was provost surgeon for southern Minnesota. In 1885 he established St. Mary's Hospital in Rochester, where his two sons later started the organization which was to become famous as the Mayo Clinic. They were both brilliant teachers, and under their leadership the Mayo Clinic rapidly became an international center for the study of surgery, William specializing in abdominal surgery and cancer, while Charles became a worldwide authority on goiter and thyroid surgery. In 1915 the brothers founded the Mayo Foundation for Medical Education and Research as a branch of the graduate school of the University of Minnesota, to which they contributed $2,800,000.

XI

The Anesthetists

THE ART OF rendering the patient unaware of pain is almost as old as illness itself. Not quite as old, however, for in the most ancient times pain was a concomitant of most forms of disease and considered a natural part of the process. The reduction of pain, or its increase, could indicate the progress of the illness and the efficacy or otherwise of the treatment being used.

There was also the idea, stemming from the early Christians, of resistance to healing of any kind, that it was purposely inflicted by God as a test or trial, and therefore all pain should be bravely borne and no attempt made to mitigate it. As was seen earlier, this attitude of mind persisted well into the nineteenth century, and in some religious sects has not vanished yet.

Despite this, throughout the centuries many attempts have been made to reduce pain and mitigate the suffering of the patient, the most obvious means being by rendering the patient insensible. The nepenthe of Homer was probably a mixture of hashish and opium, while the soporific effect of the mandrake plant was certainly known to the Assyrians. (This, incidentally, is the European mandragora and not the American mayapple of the barberry family, as is sometimes thought.) The Assyrians, too, knew of the technique of pressing on the carotid artery to produce unconsciousness, and in a later age recourse was often made to bleeding the patient until he became insensible.

Alcohol was also used for its depressant action on certain

parts of the brain, for it is not in reality a stimulant but merely retards that part of the brain that controls our less inhibited actions. The numbing effect of intense cold had been noted in the sixteenth century, and was to be rediscovered and put to a practical use by Baron Dominique Jean Larrey (1766–1842), one of Napoleon's chief surgeons, during the terrible retreat from Moscow in 1812. In India the British army surgeon James Esdaile (1749–1806) had had great success performing many operations with the patient under the influence of mesmerism, but for some reason this form of anesthesia did not become popular in England. Another old technique, revived by an Edinburgh physician, Benjamin Bell, consisted of tying a ligature around the affected limb in the hope of compressing the nerves, but this again proved unsatisfactory.

The need for a system whereby prolonged and general insensibility to pain could be induced was heightened by the increasing knowledge of the human anatomy and the longer and more complex operations that could be performed. This became more and more of an ordeal for the luckless patient. The amputation of a leg or an arm "in as little time as it takes to take a pinch of snuff" was a source of pride to many a surgeon, but operations requiring the removal of internal organs or tumors made it essential that some form of deep prolonged anesthesia should be evolved.

In the whole history of medicine few discoveries are the subject of more argument than the originator of the technique of inducing successful anesthesia. Even the inventor of the name anesthetic is in some doubt, it often being attributed to Oliver Wendell Holmes in his famous letter to Dr. William Thomas written in 1846, though the name had already been used in a paper by a London physician, John Elliotson, in 1838.

While a state of unconsciousness was a vital ingredient of any general anesthetic, the ideal product had to have far more assets than that. Insensitivity to pain was a prime requirement, but there should also be a significant degree of muscle relaxation yet at the same time complete freedom from toxicity or dangerous side effects.

The origins of modern anesthesia can probably be ascribed to

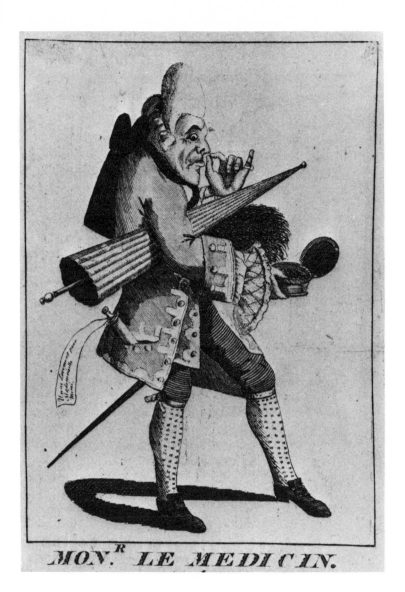

MON.ᴿ LE MEDICIN.

A French eighteenth-century cartoon showing a fashionable
"ladies doctor" of the time. The syringe is labeled
"For douching Mademoiselle Mimi."

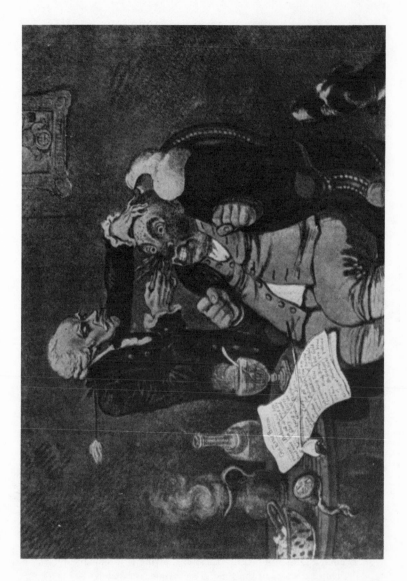

A cartoon by Gilray of a treatment with Perkins' Tractors.

the work of the Cornishman Humphry Davy (1778–1829) when employed by the eccentric Dr. Thomas Beddoes at his Medical Pneumatic Institution at Bristol. In 1799 Davy discovered the intoxicating effect of nitrous oxide, or laughing gas, and later that the same properties were found in sweet sulfuric ether, a liquid which could conveniently be carried about in small bottles. Though Davy did not pursue the matter, the news of the discovery soon crossed the Atlantic, and in the early years of the nineteenth century the social life of many doctors and researchers was enlivened by "ether frolics" on both sides of the Atlantic.

One of the most frolicsome practitioners of the time was an American country doctor, Crawford Long (1815–1878) of Jefferson, Georgia, who noticed that those who bumped themselves or sustained an injury during their frolics seemed unaware of the fact and apparently suffered no pain until the effect of the ether had worn off. He determined to put this fact to practical use, and in 1842 painlessly excised a tumor from the neck of a farm worker after first making him insensible by sniffing ether. Unfortunately, as many pioneers, Long did not appreciate the importance of his discovery to the extent of publicizing his achievement, and it was inevitable that others should eventually stumble across the same phenomenon.

One of these was a dentist, Horace Wells (1815–1848) who, in 1844 in Hartford, Connecticut, extracted the first tooth from a patient under the influence of nitrous oxide. He went on to repeat this operation several times, but his first public demonstration of an extraction under these conditions at the Massachusetts General Hospital the next year was considered to be a failure, as one of the patients groaned under the anesthetic. (Later interrogation of the patient proved that, despite this, he had felt nothing at the time.) But it was enough to discredit Wells, who thereupon turned his back on dentistry and became (of all things) a dealer in old paintings. He eventually took his own life, bitter and disillusioned, in 1848.

Amongst those present at Wells's public demonstration in 1845 was one of his former pupils, William Morton (1819–1868). He pursued his experiments with ether rather than with nitrous oxide, and a year later, at the same hospital, performed an operation painlessly and successfully before an admiring gathering of eminent medical men. But whereas Wells had not been businesslike enough, Morton went to the other extreme, disguising the chemical with aromatic herbs, giving it the name letheon and claiming its invention to himself alone. This highly unethical conduct enraged the medical profession, which was well aware that ether was the substance used, and though its advantages were confirmed, Morton himself was virtually ostracized. He made no further experiments in this field, but spent the remainder of his life in argument and litigation attempting to patent his "invention." He died of apoplexy in 1868 while driving with his wife in New York City's Central Park.

The credit for the actual discovery of anesthesia is therefore very difficult to ascribe, despite the ten thousand dollars put up by the U.S. Congress as a reward. The sum was never allocated, but as a reminder that the first public demonstrations of the technique were held in Boston, a park in that city has a monument commemorating "the discovery that the inhaling of ether causes insensibility to pain." No name of any individual is mentioned.

In Britain the first major operation using ether as an anesthetic was performed in 1846 by the eminent surgeon Robert Liston (1794–1847) at University College Hospital, London. It was for the amputation of a leg, and the doctor who actually administered the ether was Dr. Peter Squire. The operation was entirely successful, causing Liston to remark, "Gentlemen, this new Yankee dodge beats mesmerism hollow!" It also marked the beginning of the new specialty of "anesthetist" as distinct from that of surgeon or general physician.

While these notable strides forward were being made, and the use of ether was spreading throughout Europe, there were many who felt that the drug, though useful, was not an ideal substance on account of the effect its irritant properties had on many patients.

One who felt strongly on the subject was Sir James Young Simpson (1811–1870), a famous Scottish obstetrician who first used ether at a confinement in 1847. The patient, on waking from her sleep, had expressed herself refreshed and ready to undergo the pains of childbirth and at first refused to believe that her infant had already been born. So overjoyed was she when she was finally persuaded that the baby girl at her bedside was actually her own that she there and then decided to name the infant Anesthesia!

Simpson was a prime mover in the search for an alternative form of anesthetic, a search that had been going on all over Europe and America. Again, as so often happens, the answer came simultaneously from several sources. It was chloroform, discovered between 1831 and 1834 by Eugène Soubeiran in France, Samuel Guthrie in America, and Baron Justus von Liebig in Germany. A friend of Simpson, a Liverpool pharmacist named David Waldie, knew of these researches and reminded Simpson of them. Later in 1847, Simpson, Waldie, and several other friends decided to undertake a "sniffing experiment" with the new drug. Simpson was the first to awake, some time later, and, seeing the insensible bodies of his colleagues still draped around the room, decided there and then that chloroform was vastly superior to ether. Within weeks he had used chloroform in several major operations, and for the next fifty years it was to remain the drug of choice in most operations and confinements.

But the public at large did not respond with total enthusiasm to the news of this far-reaching discovery. In the somewhat smug and religiously intolerant atmosphere of the early-Victorian era, there were many who expressed themselves in opposition to any form of anesthesia, particularly in childbirth, basing their objections on the Biblical text, "I will greatly multiply thy sorrow and thy conception; in sorrow thou shalt bring forth children." (Gen. 3:16). According to these critics, Simpson and his co-workers were acting expressly against God's wishes in the matter. As one critic put it: "It would rob God of the deep, earnest cries of women in labour."

Simpson demolished these arguments in a masterly paper titled *Answers to Religious Objections Against the Employment of Anaesthetic Agents in Midwifery and Surgery* (1847) in which he demonstrated as intimate a knowledge of the Bible as he had of human anatomy. Indeed, he turned the tables on his critics by also quoting from Genesis 2:21 to prove that God Himself had undertaken an operation under anesthesia, in the passage, "And the Lord caused a deep sleep to fall upon Adam, and he slept: and he took one of his ribs and closed up the flesh instead thereof."

However, despite these religious and moral arguments, much was done to make anesthesia in childbirth fashionable when Queen Victoria herself agreed to its use on the occasion of the birth of her eighth child in 1853. Opposition finally crumbled when she used it again for her next and last confinement, that of Princess Beatrice, in 1857. For some years afterward childbirth anesthesia was known as anesthesia *a la reine*.

The first full-time professional anesthetist was Dr. John Snow, the same doctor who proved that cholera was spread by contaminated water. It was he who administered the anesthesia to Queen Victoria. By the time he died, he was assisting in over four hundred operations a year.

While chloroform or chloroform-and-ether mixtures were finding increasing favor in Europe and America, an American chemist, Gardner Colton (1814–1898), had steadfastly continued his experiments with nitrous oxide. In partnership with a dentist friend, he demonstrated the complete success of nitrous oxide in dental extractions, traveling all over the country, and in 1863, with another partner, Dr. John Smith, opened the Colton Dental Association in New York.

Early in 1869, Professor E. Andrews of Chicago began using a mixture of oxygen and nitrous oxide to prolong anesthesia, a technique which rapidly found favor in England where pure nitrous oxide had never become so generally popular as in America because of its side effects.

Gradually the use of different anesthetics became associated with different kinds of operations, nitrous oxide becoming popular for dentistry, while ether or chloroform was used almost exclusively for major operations. But even the use of chloroform became a subject of criticism and discussion by reason of the occasional fatalities that occurred during its use, some no doubt due to the drug itself, but others presumably due to the surgery.

Simpson, for example, maintained that death under chloroform was usually due to respiratory failure, and therefore that the drug should be used simply and sparingly, with no more than a soaked handkerchief or towel pressed to the nostrils. Snow, on the other hand, insisted that uncontrolled amounts of chloroform affected the heart, and that a precise and carefully regulated dose should be administered, preferably by means of an instrument he himself had invented. He also maintained that the state of the patient's pulse should be checked throughout the operation.

In 1875 the British Medical Association inaugurated a commission to investigate the matter. It took five years to publicize its findings, which were that chloroform was much more injurious to the heart than nitrous oxide or ether. In 1889 the wealthy nizam of Hyderabad financed a further series of tests in India which concluded that, in a series of experiments on dogs, heart failure took place only *after* respiratory failure. Not to be outdone, the B.M.A. immediately mounted another commission which this time took ten years to inform the waiting world that no definite conclusions had been reached. Yet another inquiry was started in 1901, the Special Chloroform Commission, which in 1911 was able to report that a 2 percent concentration of chloroform in air was the ideal mixture, enough to anesthetize sufficiently yet not enough to damage the heart. It also recommended the use of a special inhaler to regulate the concentration.

Side by side with the search for a suitable product capable of producing general anesthesia, some physicians had concerned themselves with the problem of discovering a local, or surface, anesthetic. There had been hints of the existence of such a product far back in antiquity. Homer, in Book II of the *Iliad,* mentioned a bitter root which, when applied to a wound, "took pain away and ended all anguish." Dioscorides, in the first century A.D., had ascribed similar attributes to a substance called "Memphian Stone" (possibly a type of marble). In 1530 the Conquistadores had brought back from Peru news of a wonderful plant called coca which was first described in English by Dr. John Frampton in his pleasantly titled book, *Joyfull Newes out of the Newe Founde Worlde* (1577).

By the end of the eighteenth century, supplies of this plant were reaching Europe in quantity and by 1859 pharmacology had progressed to the extent that a German chemist, Albert Neimann, had isolated the active ingredient of the plant, the alkaloid cocaine. Various experiments with it were conducted in different countries, and as early as 1869 cocaine was being used as a local anesthetic by the famous French ear, nose, and throat specialist, Charles Flauvel. By 1884 others were also investigating its use, notably H. J. Knapp of New York (1831–1911).

Cocaine is, admittedly, a highly dangerous and habit-forming drug, and for most of the twentieth century the search has continued for equally effective but less toxic drugs resulting in the emergence of substances like lignocaine, cinchocaine, betamethasone, and mepyramine maleate, all intended for topical or surface use. Certain local anesthetics are injected spinally for operations on the lower limbs, but in the majority of more serious operations involving the body cavities, general anesthetics continue to be used.

One important aspect of anesthesia is the use of muscle relaxants which cause the limbs to be manipulated more easily and which aid the surgeon. This too, has a long history. Part of the "Joyfull Newes" of John Frampton in 1577 was the report of the discovery of the South American arrow poison curare, of which tobacco was said to be an antidote, and to be described later by the Victorian explorer Waterton.

In 1745 the first dried samples of curare were investigated in Paris and in Leyden, and in 1781 the French doctor/priest, the Abbé Fontana, demonstrated that the drug, though paralyzing respiration when injected, was harmless when swallowed and did not affect the heart.

In 1859, Sir Thomas Spencer Wells (1818–1897) first used curare in the treatment of lockjaw, and it continued to be used for epilepsy, chorea, and hydrophobia, all diseases where severe convulsions are a feature and muscular spasms need to be controlled or modified. Because of the particular effect of curare on the respiratory system, it has been of value in studying the effects of inhaled anesthetics such as chloroform and ether and so led to more modern products such as halothane.

Present research is also much concerned with the production

of anesthetics which will cause fewer side effects and be rapidly expelled from the body. In the long-term, chemically induced anesthesia may be replaced or supplemented by other means, such as hypnosis, or by electrical treatment which interferes with the transmission of nerve impulses. There will always be a risk in such experimentation, but following in the steps of Simpson and others, there will always be doctors ready to investigate the method of anesthesia and try it out on themselves, so guiding the researchers along the most hopeful lines. If there is one thing that is not dormant it is anesthesia.

XII

Microbe Men

No NATURAL FUNCTION which the human male experiences during the course of his life is as traumatic as what a woman goes through in the delivery of a child. Yet the early history of medicine and illness shows that though childbirth was never, at its best, a comfortable process even under natural conditions, it was rarely attended by any great danger to the mother. It seems therefore something of a paradox that danger to the mother resulting from puerperal fever should have coincided with the custom, beginning in the sixteenth century, of the physician attending confinements, rather than the midwife. As time went on the development of hospitals and the increased use of lying-in wards appeared to aggravate the situation rather than improve it.

Puerperal fever had been noted as a risk attending the birth of a child from ancient times, but never on a large scale. From the sixteenth century onward it increased in intensity, and between 1650 and 1850 Europe was ravaged by some two hundred epidemics of the disease, the worst being in 1773 in the Lombardy region of Italy when, during the course of twelve months, not one woman lived after delivering her child. Doctors and surgeons were completely at a loss in establishing the cause, the most common theory being that it was something to do with the weather. This took no account of the fact that women giving birth in their own homes were much less likely to contract the illness than those confined in hospitals, though the hospital was intended to provide care and comfort and to ease the pangs of labor.

This was the situation at the beginning of the nineteenth century when the New Viennese School of Medicine was at its height and represented the vanguard of modern medical thought and progress throughout the whole of Europe.

Like other great hospitals the Allgemeine Krankenhaus (People's Hospital) of Vienna had its own lying-in departments, and in 1845 the first assistant in the maternity wards was Ignaz Philipp Semmelweiss (1818–1865). An observant man, he noticed that there was a great disparity in the incidence of puerperal fever in the two wards under his control. In the ward supervised almost entirely by nurses and midwives, mortality remained at a fairly constant figure of 3 percent. But in the ward which was used for the instruction of medical students, and where they physically examined the patients in the course of their studies, mortality averaged 18 percent and occasionally reached 30 percent.

This curious fact did not pass unnoticed by the women of Vienna who were brought to the hospital for confinement, many of them prostitutes off the street, who fought strenuously to be confined in the ward staffed by midwives and not in the ward attended by students. Semmelweiss, too, worried over this matter, though he was at first the only physician in the hospital to do so. The constant arrival of the priest, coming to give the Last Sacraments to the dying women, presented a challenge to him that he knew he must meet. Later he was to comment: "It was a fresh shock to me every time I heard the bell as the priest passed my door, and once again I heaved a sigh for the victim who was to be destroyed by an unknown cause. The bell, in fact, became for me an exhortation to search with all my energies to elucidate the cause."

In 1847 he stumbled upon a clue. In that year his great friend and colleague Kolletscha died from an infection sustained by pricking his finger at a postmortem. Semmelweiss noticed that the symptoms of the fever that preceded his death bore a marked resemblance to the symptoms of puerperal fever. Immediately the association between postmortems undertaken by the students and their subsequent examination of pregnant women came to mind. The students came straight from the dissecting rooms, where they had been handling corpses, and without any washing of hands or other precaution, immediately began to examine the pregnant women. It seemed very likely that the answer to the problem lay here.

He immediately installed a routine by which every student coming from the dissecting rooms had first to wash his hands in a solution of chloride of lime before entering the maternity wards. The result was startling. Within a week the incidence of puerperal fever in the students' ward dropped to 3 percent, the same as in the other ward, and very soon reduced to 1 percent. Semmelweiss had found the answer, and excitedly reported to the hospital authorities, "Puerperal fever is caused by conveyance to the pregnant woman of putrid particles derived from living organisms, through the agency of the examining fingers."

It might be thought that this all-important discovery would be welcomed by his contemporaries as a significant forward step, but it was not to be. His superiors at the hospital put it down to coincidence and insisted that puerperal fever was a natural phenomenon and a normal risk of childbirth. The difference in the mortality rate of the two wards, they said, was due to the fact that the "finer feelings" of the women examined by the students was disturbed by the presence of men. As the majority of patients in this ward were prostitutes, this hardly seemed to be a workable theory.

Semmelweiss, never one to suffer fools gladly, barked back at his critics. Writing to the famous German obstetrician, Paul Scanzoni, who ridiculed his ideas, Semmelweiss accused him of the indiscriminate murder of thousands of women by not accepting his findings, and called him "a medical Nero." Even in the backbiting context of normal correspondence between eminent doctors, this was going too far, and in 1851 Semmelweiss resigned from the Vienna hospital and returned to his native Budapest. There he put his theories into practice at the hospital of St. Rochus, where conditions had been even more primitive than in Vienna, and where the mortality rate was reduced even more dramatically on his arrival.

Yet while Semmelweiss was suffering from this violent opposition to what seemed a logical theory, in other parts of Europe surgeons, and obstetricians in particular, were coming to appreciate the value of absolute cleanliness in operations, though the reasons for it were by no means apparent. In London, Sir Thomas Spencer Wells, the most eminent surgeon and early pioneer in the removal of ovarian tumors, had an astonishingly high success rate which he attributed to his absolute insistence on cleanliness. Nearly fifty years earlier Alexander Gordon of Aberdeen, in a long-forgotten paper, had advocated the fumigation of all instruments before an operation or confinement. In Boston, Massachusetts, in 1842, Oliver Wendell Holmes, perhaps better known as a man of letters than a physician, had been howled down by his audience when he read a paper on "The Contagiousness of Puerperal Fever" and had recommended a complete change of clothing before conducting a confinement. His reply to his critics was a pertinent one. "Medical logic," he observed, "does not appear to be taught or practiced in our medical schools." This was indeed true, and Semmelweiss was to pay for it. The lack of acceptance of his ideas on hygiene eventually preyed on his mind, and he was at last forced to enter an asylum where he died in 1865.

Two close contemporaries of Semmelweiss were, in the end, to vindicate the validity of his theories and to open the door to the acceptance of the theory of germ infection. In France it was not a doctor who carried out this work, but a brilliant chemist, Louis Pasteur (1822–1895), while in England the physician Joseph Lister (1827–1912) made his own significant contribution.

Pasteur was born in the Jura, a wine-growing district of France, and after taking his examinations became assistant to Dumas, the professor of chemistry at the Ecole Normale in Paris. There his first piece of original work was in the structure of tartaric acid, where he demonstrated that two forms existed, identical in formula, but behaving differently under polarized light. This research on the levorotatory and dextrorotatory attributes of certain chemicals was to lay the foundations of stereochemistry.

But it was in his research into the behavior of alcohol that Pasteur made his most significant contribution to medicine. In

1854 he was appointed professor of chemistry at Lille, in the north of France, a city which though not in a wine-growing area was very largely concerned with the behavior of alcohol in the form of beer.

Pasteur noted that both beer and wine seemed to "fall sick" after being stored for a short time, and after much experimentation he evolved the technique of heating the liquids and then allowing them to cool. By this means they retained their original purity and the system of Pasteurization was born. But more importantly he demonstrated that ferments and alcoholic solutions were not affected if fresh air was not allowed to reach them. In the presence of air he noted that many chemical substances seemed to be transformed into other chemicals—lactose became lactic acid, butter fat became butyric acid, and so on. As these changes took place only if the original chemical was exposed to air, and not if they were hermetically sealed, it seemed logical to suppose that the change was brought about by microorganisms floating in the atmosphere and invisible to the naked eye.

He extended this theory to the study of airborne organisms which might induce chemical changes in the body, and so precipitate disease. Going back to the work of Jenner and his vaccination against smallpox by deliberately inducing a modified form of the disease to prevent a serious outbreak, he extended this theory to the treatment of anthrax and chicken cholera, two diseases which, at the time, were having serious repercussions on French farming.

His most famous experiments, however, were in the control of hydrophobia in man. In 1885 he treated his first case of rabies with a vaccine made from the dehydrated spine of a rabid dog, and later that year was completely successful in treating a young boy, Jean-Baptiste Jupille, who had bravely wrestled with a mad dog in order to protect his younger companions. A statue commemorating the bravery of the boy stands outside the Pasteur Institute in Paris today. The institute was first opened in 1888, and the treatment of six Russian peasants there suspected of suffering from hydrophobia after being mauled by a pack of rabid wolves is dramatically described by the Swedish doctor, Axel Munthe, in his book, *The Story of San Michele*.

With Pasteur's further experiments in bacteriology, including his saving of the French silkworm industry by arresting an epidemic, it can readily be appreciated how this great chemist's contribution to industry, medicine, and agriculture have resulted in a Rue Pasteur being found in virtually every town and city throughout France.

In Scotland, soon after the death of Semmelweiss, an English-born doctor was also concerning himself with diseases found mainly in hospitals. Joseph Lister was born near London, in Essex, in 1827, qualified as a surgeon at University College in the capital, and in 1860 was appointed regius professor of surgery in Glasgow. Infection within the hospital had been rife for some time, but was thought to be due to faulty drains, and poisonous gases or "miasmas" emanating from sewers and cesspits. To counteract the high degree of infection existing, it was thought that all that could be done was to wash the instruments and the hands of the operator in cold boiled water, a process which did little to solve the problem.

Surgeons of the time habitually operated in frock coats, with no other protective clothing, the coats being so encrusted with dried blood and pus from innumerable operations that the garment became rigid enough to be capable of standing erect on its own. For many surgeons this had become almost a status symbol, for the formation of pus in a wound had for centuries been considered "laudable" and a perfectly natural and normal phenomenon.

Like Semmelweiss, Joseph Lister worried about the presence of hospital "miasmas" and the high incidence of infection after operations of all kinds. He considered that if a miasma really existed, it was more likely to be not a fog but an exceedingly fine form of pollen floating in the atmosphere. He, too, arrived at the conclusion that it was the air that caused the trouble, and based this on his observation of the difference between simple and compound fractures. In a simple fracture, where the bone was broken within the limb and had not pierced the surrounding flesh, no pus formed at the site of the fracture. But in a compound fracture, where the bone end protruded through the flesh and exposed the wound to the air, infection was the almost inevitable consequence. Indeed, infection was so common under these conditions that in amputations the rate of mortality was between 30 percent and 50 percent.

Lister decided that in the absence of any means of reducing the "pollen" in the atmosphere, the next best thing was to try and neutralize it at the site. He therefore cast around for some chemical that might achieve this, and remembered that a Manchester chemist named Calvert had reported success in using carbolic acid to disinfect and deodorize sewage and excreta in cesspits. Lister decided to experiment with this substance, and in March 1865 first used carbolic acid on a compound fracture, soaking in the solution the wound, the dressings, and even the hands of the operator and nurses. No infection occurred and the operation was completely successful. Lister then invented a special form of atomizer with which all surfaces, instruments, hands, and clothing were sprayed with carbolic before every operation. This form of spray became standard procedure for many years in Scottish hospitals.

In that same year of 1865, which also saw the tragic death of Semmelweiss, Lister first heard of the work of Pasteur and knew that he was working on the right lines.

Though Lister's theories were accepted in Scotland, English surgeons were much slower to follow, and it was in Germany that his ideas found the readiest acceptance. The benefits of this were seen in the hygiene regulations affecting field hospitals of the German army in their victory over the French in the Franco-Prussian War of 1870–1871. Acceptance was also slow in America, and as late as 1882 Lister was still being attacked at meetings of the American Surgical Association.

Lister's attention to detail was the basis of his success, and his ideas were put to work in many facets of operational technique. He introduced the catgut ligature and showed how to sterilize it, and pioneered the use of sinus forceps and probe-pointed scissors. He popularized the use of the rubber drainage-tube in operations, evolved by the French surgeon Pierre Chassaignac in 1867, and first employed it in the course of a minor operation on Queen Victoria in 1871 at Balmoral, Scotland.

In 1883, Joseph Lister became Lord Lister, the first British surgeon to be raised to the peerage. From 1865 he had corresponded closely with Pasteur, and the two eminent men became firm friends. When Lister died in 1912 at the age of eighty-five the Royal College of Physicians, in their eulogy, said, "His work will last for all time; humanity will bless him evermore and his fame will be immortal."

Pasteur and Lister, though at first working independently, formulated the theory of germ-borne disease, Lister becoming the apostle of antisepsis (the killing of bacteria) and later of asepsis (the stopping of the formation of bacteria). It was left to a German doctor, Robert Koch (1843–1910), to take the work a stage further and to attempt to identify and classify the various kinds of germs present in the atmosphere, and so found the science of bacteriology.

Koch was a comparatively young man of twenty-nine when he was first appointed medical officer of the small town of Bomst in Germany. He was a keen and observant scientist, and in this large rural area was concerned about the constant outbreaks of splenic fever, now called anthrax, which affected the livestock and was so easily transmitted to humans. He went back to the original work of a German veterinarian, Franz Pollender, who, in 1849, had examined the blood of anthrax victims through a microscope and had discovered the presence of a number of rod-like organisms in the blood. Koch experimented further, and found that these organisms, which were the bacilli of anthrax, propagated themselves by transverse fission to form spores. These spores, when passed through the animal and liberated into the atmosphere, remained virulent for many years and were resistant to all known forms of antiseptic. This explained why, though individual cases of anthrax could be cured and alleviated, further epidemics were constantly occurring.

Koch, as so many had done before him, returned to the work of Jenner and his theory of attenuated vaccines, artificially cultivating anthrax spores in the laboratory, diluting the culture, and injecting the vaccine. As was expected a comparatively minor outbreak of anthrax was precipitated, enabling the body to activate what appeared to be some form of defense mechanism which, in this case, gave lifelong immunity. Other workers followed his lead, and gradually other bacilli were isolated, including those of gonorrhea, typhoid, and leprosy.

Koch himself pursued his studies in the field of wounds and the isolation of bacteria causing infection. In 1882 he discovered the tubercle bacillus, proving that consumption was not, as was thought, a wasting disease caused by malnutrition but an infectious disease transferable to others.

Probably his most important discovery was of the cholera, or the comma, bacillus which had created such devastation in Europe and America in at least three outbreaks since 1822. He found that the disease was sparked off by infected water-supplies, and his researches in this field enabled a whole range of diseases to be controlled, if not eliminated.

If Koch's work did not result in the absolute extermination of epidemics it did, at least, point the way by which future researchers should be guided. A vital step forward was made by one of his pupils, Emil von Behring (1854–1917), who discovered the means by which the defense mechanism of the body dealt with bacteria-induced disease.

Behring discovered that certain bacilli, when introduced into the body, produced albuminous organisms called toxins, and it was these toxins which actually caused the disease. The human body counteracted this by producing further organisms called antitoxins, which combined with the toxins and neutralized them. Unfortunately it frequently happened that the invasion of bacteria, and the production of toxins, was so rapid that the body did not have time to produce the requisite number of antitoxins and illness resulted and the disease ran its course. Behring argued that if the antitoxins of, say, diphtheria, which had been formed in the blood serum of an animal, were injected into a human being, this would augment the body's own store of antitoxins and immunity would result. Further, if diphtheria were already present in the human body, the added antitoxins would immediately neutralize it. This proved to be the case, and the study of this phenomenon and the use of antitoxins in a wide range of diseases has now become the science of immunology. Thanks to Behring, following in the footsteps of Jenner, Lister, and Pasteur, diphtheria, once the scourge of the infant population, is now almost unknown. Tetanus antitoxin has effectively reduced the high danger of infection and death from open wounds.

In America much valuable work in the same field was done by Theobald Smith (1859–1934), a physician whose main contribution to bacteriology was in the differentiation of avian, bovine, and human tubercle bacilli, in the treatment of Texas fever in cattle, and in his original work on the mechanism of allergies. He was the first director of the State Laboratory of Massachusetts in 1895 and went on to become the first professor of comparative pathology at Harvard. His colleague William Welch (1850–1934) discovered the bacillus of gas grangrene in 1892, but later gave up bacteriology for the study of medical history. His memorial is the Institute of Medical History and the Welch Medical Library, both in Baltimore.

Emil Behring himself was awarded the Nobel Prize for Medicine in 1901. He would have been the first to admit that his success was due very largely to the sure foundation laid down by those "germ doctors" who had gone before.

XIII

The Evolution of the Alienists

"THE BRAIN IS the organ where madness is born," said Hippocrates, so providing an honorable ancestry to the contention that mental illness is due to some malfunction of part of the body. Yet for a considerable time this was not the accepted view. Madness, which frequently appeared to have no connection with any other bodily disorder or symptom, was more easily diagnosed as "possession" by evil spirits, at a time when illness of any kind, mental or physical, was judged to be a punishment from the gods for some transgression, or a departure from the normal code of conduct.

Primitive man attempted to rid sufferers of the evil spirits by exorcism and extraordinary rites and rituals performed by the village witch doctor. Among the North American Indians, the witch doctors always included a specialist in demonic possession, called a shaman, who himself must have undergone some traumatic emotional mental disturbance before he could be officially appointed.

In some communities, if exorcism failed, the luckless victim was buried alive in the hope that the malevolent spirit would be entombed with him and unable to escape and affect other members of the community.

Of the ancient medical writers, only the Greek doctor Soranus recognized the possible causes of madness, and attempted to treat victims by sympathy and understanding. Though it was more than a thousand years before his ideas were to be studied again, Soranus can thus be credited with being the first, if remote, student of psychiatry in its modern meaning.

For the general mass of the people and their physicians, madness was still considered to be possession by the devil, and in the early Christian era to be attributed to the mad person's having dabbled in magic and witchcraft. The first official burning of a witch took place in A.D. 430, but the real battle against witchcraft did not make itself felt for many years, until the rising tide of "magic" in Europe forced the church to act.

This it did in 1484 when Pope Innocent VIII issued a papal bull in which anyone engaged in magic or necromancy was branded as a heretic and excommunicated. The result was immediate and terrible. Once given power to take action against witches, the clergy throughout Europe unleashed their pent-up venom in an orgy of persecution and torture which was to last the best part of three hundred years, and during which an estimated million supposed witches were to be put to death.

The "bible" of the clergy in this matter was a book called the *Malleus Maleficarum* (Hammer of the Witches), written by two monks of Cologne, Jacobus Sprenger and Heinrich Kramer, in 1486, two years after the bull. They gave themselves the title of "Domini canes" or Hounds of the Lord, and were members of the Dominican Order. Not only did they fulminate against witchcraft in any form, but provided guidelines by which those dabbling in magic, or possessed, could be identified. In the final portion of the book, exact and explicit instructions were given on how to extract confessions by torture and how to deal with those who were convicted.

In fact the outlook for any alleged witch (mostly women and girls) was bleak in the extreme. It usually began by gossip in the village, perhaps through a child suffering from epilepsy, or a woman said to have the "evil eye" and supposedly causing a spinning machine to stop or milk to curdle. Even in the preliminary trial at village level, the dice was already loaded against the witch, for a favorite test was to bind her hands and feet and throw her into the pond or river. If she floated she was guilty, and immediately handed over to the official witchcraft court, but if she sank, and very probably drowned, she was considered innocent!

Once in the hands of the inquisitors at the special court, her fate was sealed. Torture was used to extract a full "confession" and to elicit the names of other known witches in the community. Once her guilt had been proved, and she had confessed, another series of tortures began as a penalty for her sins against God and the Church. Should the victim survive these prolonged agonies, she was finally publicly burned at the stake, an end which for most must have been a happy release.

Though witches were dealt with in this way, it was already becoming to be recognized in the Middle Ages that not all madness could be attributed to possession. In England, as distinct from other European countries such as Germany and Spain, there was a greater degree of tolerance. Probably the first hospital especially allocated to the housing of the insane was the Bethlem (or Bedlam) Hospital in London which received its first insane patient in 1377, though it had been a conventional hospital since 1247.

Restraint was the keynote of all treatment for the mentally afflicted, and the equipment of Bedlam consisted of huge numbers of chains, rings, padlocks, fetters, and cages in which the patients were confined. For many centuries, until the early 1800s, a favorite Sunday afternoon excursion for Londoners was to visit the Bedlam Hospital to watch the antics of the inmates and to goad them into even greater frenzies.

The first modern research into madness was conducted by a German doctor, Johann Wyer (1515–1588), who realized that those said to be possessed were in reality suffering from some kind of mental affliction, and that their actions and hallucinations were due to this and not, of necessity, caused by the devil. He was also the first doctor to investigate the phenomenon of mass hysteria and hallucinations, the causes of which modern psychiatrists are still attempting to find.

In England another doctor, Reginald Scot (1538–1599), was also investigating madness and coming much to the same conclusions as Wyer in Germany. In 1584 Scot published his book on the subject, which immediately sparked off a counterblast from no less a personage than King James VI of Scotland. The king, in his famous *Demonology*, insisted that witchcraft was the basic and underlying reason for almost any kind of evil behavior.

In Switzerland the eminent physician Felix Plater (1536–1614) had also studied insanity, but though he visited the inmates in their dungeon cells and took the trouble to dissect the corpses of over three hundred insane persons, he could not rid himself of the idea that madness was the work of the devil.

As the witchcraft hysteria in Europe gradually died down, doctors developed a more rational attitude toward mental ills, though in some instances their theories seemed almost as bizarre as the earlier beliefs. In 1765, for example, a French physician, Jean-Pierre Grosley, had decided that out of all the countries in Europe, England had the highest incidence of "lunatics and madmen" due, he said, to the national fondness for beer and roast beef. He was also of the opinion that England was a nation of potential suicides brought about by living in the murky atmosphere of fogs which most foreigners believed plunged England into an impenetrable gloom from January to December. He dubbed melancholia "the English Malady," very likely to get his own back for the English habit of referring to syphilis as "the French Disease."

The second half of the eighteenth century was marked by the rapid rise of the hydro or spa in Europe and in America as a means of curing every imaginable ailment. So popular did this treatment become that Horace Walpole was constrained to remark that "the English must be descended from a race of ducks, the speed with which they take to the water." A session at a spa was particularly popular for treatment of supposed madness and hysteria, and for ladies of "a nervous disposition," but judging from some of the goings-on at Bath, Matlock, and other well-known hydros, most ladies had reason to be more nervous after they arrived than before. But when George III decided to try the seaside air of Weymouth, on the south coast, the custom of bathing, both inland or at the seaside, became more respectable.

A Dr. William Falconer of Bath wrote a bestselling book in 1790 on *The Medicinal Properties of Bath Water*, which he dedicated to George III in the hope that he might come to Bath should he have a relapse from the attack of madness which had created such problems for the government in 1788 and 1789.

The medical history of George III has been a source of confusion to historians on both sides of the Atlantic for nearly two hundred years. In 1855 *The Times* of London, unfortunately taken by most countries to reflect the official attitude of the British government, which it rarely did, carried an article which said, slightly spitefully: "Our Transatlantic brethren may probably trace in the results of the mental disorder of George III, their own elevation to national status."

In fact nobody could trace the elevation of the American people to national status from this cause, for the very good reason that the first mental derangement of the king, now known to be due to a disease called porphyria, did not occur until 1788, twelve years after the Declaration of Independence. But the result of this attack, and the gradual deterioration of the king's mental powers from 1801 until his death in 1820, have had the effect of coloring retrospectively all the actions of the king during the earlier part of his reign. The disease from which the king suffered is due to a metabolic disturbance which has the effect of increasing the pigmented organisms in the bloodstream called porphyrins. This results in an acute skin sensitivity to sunlight, with a corresponding rash, wine-colored urine in many cases, and in its extreme form with intermittent mental derangement and melancholy. Though the king had had a short outbreak of porphyria in 1765, when he was twenty-six years old, there is no evidence that this affected him mentally. During the whole of his long reign (he died in his eighty-second year), his madness, for want of a better word, amounted to a total of just over six months and did not begin until he was fifty years of age. From 1810 to 1820 Britain was under the prince regent, later George IV.

It was during the reign of George III that the first experiments were made in freeing lunatics from restraint and, as so often happens with experiments, they took place in different countries independently.

In France the well-known Paris doctor Philippe Pinel (1745–1826) had been appointed to the huge Bicêtre mental hospital.

What he discovered there shocked him profoundly. He found that patients had been manacled and chained to their beds, sometimes for years on end, with scarcely a chance to move a limb and certainly no opportunity to walk about, and he determined to put an end to this inhuman form of treatment. In 1792 he wrote an important paper outlining his theories on the treatment of the insane, A *Medico-Philosophical Treatise on Mental Alienation,* but because of the upheaval caused by the French Revolution, this was not published until 1801, though he was grudgingly allowed to put his ideas into practice as soon as he was appointed to the Bicêtre. On at least one occasion his ideas were thought to be so dangerous that he was in danger of being attacked by the mob, and had to be rescued by his own "insane" patients!

During this same period, and at a time when communication between England and France was difficult, similar conclusions had been arrived at by a Quaker merchant named William Tuke (1732–1822), a resident of the city of York. In 1792, shocked by the revelations of the treatment meted out to patients in the York County Asylum, he persuaded the local members of the Society of Friends to raise funds for the building of a special mental hospital in the county for private use. This was called The Retreat and was completed and in business by 1796. Tuke, of course, had no knowledge of the work of Pinel in France at the time.

By far the worst conditions were in the notorious Bedlam Hospital in London where it was discovered that an American inmate, James Norris, had not only been chained to his bed for over twelve years, but during all this time he had had an iron collar around his neck fixed to an upright pole at the bedhead.

At the York County Asylum the situation had been much improved by an ingenious ploy on the part of the local Quakers. At the annual general meeting, Tuke and his friends had appeared in force, and ten of them had each subscribed fifty dollars, thus automatically becoming governors and outvoting the existing management.

But in the country as a whole, though the situation was being investigated, there was little compulsion on the part of the municipal authorities to improve conditions in their asylums. Few towns had such enlightened and generous citizens as York, while those that did, like Bristol, were more concerned with the conditions in the prisons and penal institutions than in the local madhouses.

In 1828, Dr. John Conolly (1794–1866) had attempted to preach the gospel against restraining lunatics, at University College Hospital in London. There were few who took any notice, and in 1839 he applied for, and obtained, a position at one of England's largest asylums, that at Hanwell, Middlesex, a few miles west of London. It was Conolly, in his official position, together with Tuke and his friends in York, and Edward Charlesworth and Robert Hall, physicians of Lincoln, who made the government enforce reforms.

Similar progress was being made in France, where Pinel was followed at the Bicêtre by Dr. Jean-Dominique Esquirol (1722–1840) and Guillaume Ferrus (1784–1861). Both these physicians contributed greatly to the founding of modern psychiatric methods, Esquirol by his famous textbook *On Mental Illness* (1838) and Ferrus by insisting that the government should provide a home farm at all mental institutions, so inaugurating the concept of occupational therapy in the treatment of the insane.

In America equally important work was being done by a woman, Dorothea Lynde Dix (1802–1887), a schoolmistress, philanthropist, and social reformer who worked tirelessly to improve the lot of paupers, prisoners, and lunatics. In 1848 she reported to Congress that she had personally visited and interviewed nearly ten thousand lunatics and epileptics in various institutions up and down the country and found the majority bound and manacled and treated in the most shocking manner. As a result of her work, over thirty new mental hospitals were built in the years that followed, and the conditions in the others immeasurably improved. The basic assumption of Dorothea Dix was that the insane could be cured by "moral treatment." This was the belief that comfortable and cheerful surroundings and kindness could permanently improve the lot of the insane and bring about a cure. This had worked well enough when the patients were middle and upper middle class and in private institutions. At such well-known places as the Bloomingdale Asylum in New York, the Pennsylvania Hospital in Philadelphia, and the Hartford Retreat in Connecticut, it was found that over half the patients responded.

Unfortunately in the new state institutions for the insane poor for which Dorothea Dix had fought, the results were nowhere near as good. The "moral treatment" depended on the doctor and the patient sharing the same cultural values. And communication broke down completely between the very poor—often of immigrant background—and the doctors. In addition the institutions became so crowded that little more than custodial care could be done. Gradually the treatment promoted so enthusiastically by Dorothea Dix became outmoded and a new theory was evolved—that insanity was almost certainly genetic in origin and could therefore not be cured. The result of this pessimistic attitude was that though the insane were no longer restrained and treated cruelly, little was done in the way of active therapeutic treatment for them. This was to be the attitude for the remainder of the nineteenth century.

After her work among the insane Dorothea Dix was appointed superintendent of nursing services during the Civil War. She had to combat the entrenched antagonism of the male physicians, but nevertheless was instrumental in bringing about some notable reforms in the nursing profession. Though a zealous reformer, she was no administrator and at the end of the Civil War was passed over by the government when civilian posts were being allocated. Somewhat disillusioned, she withdrew from the world of nursing and medicine and returned to her earlier hobby of writing books for children.

During this period, in England much thought had been given to the question of the responsibility of those who were insane but who had committed crimes. As the result of a famous case in 1828, when a lunatic named Bellingham had shot and killed the British prime minister, many doubts had been raised as to the justice of executing a man for a crime committed when he was manifestly out of his mind, and had been for some time. The matter came to a head a few years later, in 1843, when a man called Daniel McNaghten tried to shoot another British prime minister, this time Sir Robert Peel, but shot and killed his secretary instead. The defense of McNaghten was that he was suffering from an acute persecution mania, enough to turn his mind, and was not responsible for his actions. As the result of intervention by the House of Lords, the McNaghten Rules were formulated, specifying that a man could not be convicted of a crime if, at the time, he was suffering from such a defect of reason that he was unaware of what he was doing, or that he was doing wrong, or that he was unaware of the consequences of his action. McNaghten, whose state of mind fulfilled these conditions, was therefore not condemned to death but sent to an asylum.

As a result of the formulation of the McNaghten Rules, other criminals and murderers were reprieved during the next few years.

From the middle of the nineteenth century, though the ideas of Anton Mesmer had been largely discredited as a source of universal healing, experiments were revived in the use of hypnosis, particularly in the treatment of the nervous or hysterical patient. The most notable work in this field had been done by Jean Charcot (1825–1893), senior neurologist at the Salpêtrière, the great hospital in Paris for the nervous diseases of women. There, together with his pupil Hypolite Bernheim (1840–1919), he had used hypnosis in the treatment of the paralysis of the insane.

In Vienna, and later in Paris with Charcot, Sigmund Freud (1856–1939) claimed even more success and longer-lasting results by interrogating his patients under hypnosis, making them reveal their subconscious fears and desires and tracing this back to their early infant and childhood experiences. From this technique, described as "mental catharsis," and from the analysis of dreams, Freud became the founder of modern psychoanalysis.

Freud had qualified as a doctor in 1881 and his first medical researches had been in the use of cocaine. In this he was doomed to failure, chiefly on account of the serious drawbacks to cocaine because of its addictive properties. As he himself said: "I have very restricted capacities or talents. None at all for the natural sciences; nothing for mathematics; nothing for anything quantitative." Freud's strength lay in his ability to see behind the workings of the human mind and in his intensely imaginative approach to this work. He was also an inspiration to others working in the same field.

In Vienna, contemporary with Freud, a brilliant young doctor, Josef Breuer (1842–1925), had also been experimenting with hypnosis. Together the two men evolved the concept that all neuroses are due to suppressed sexual desires, including incest— ideas which came as a cold and unpalatable douche to the majority of neurologists in Europe at the time.

Also associated with Freud and Breuer in Vienna was another doctor, Alfred Adler (1870–1937), who was the first of Freud's disciples to break away from him. Adler insisted that it was not repressed sexuality that caused neuroses, but the repressed desire to dominate and triumph over others. This was the reason, he said, for the headaches, illnesses, and even partial paralysis of many people, which merely demonstrated their subconscious attempt to make everyone subservient to them and willing to do their bidding. Adler created his own School of Individual Psychology, and was the instigator of the theory of the inferiority complex.

Another of Freud's associates was the Swiss physician, Carl Gustav Jung (1875–1961), who, though at first accepting Freud's theories, soon went off on his own path after their first meeting in 1912. For Jung it was the will to live which created neuroses, and he differed from Freud in believing that these could be resolved by analyzing the existing problems and maladjustments of patients rather than going back into their past lives and revealing their repressed sexual and infantile fantasies. These ideas Jung formulated as the basis of his School of Analytical Psychology.

Today, modern psychoanalysts use the ideas of all three men, Freud, Adler, and Jung, and many new theories are still being evolved. But in many countries many practicing physicians still consider psychoanalysis to be slightly suspect, and anyone seeking the services of a psychiatrist is in danger of being thought a little mad. As the late Samuel Goldwyn is said to have commented, "Anyone who goes to a psychiatrist ought to have his head examined!"

In comparison with the revolutionary advances made in

medicine during the nineteenth century, it is only during the twentieth century that psychiatry has really come into its own. Though Freud and his disciples concentrated chiefly on the workings of the "subconscious," they had no illusions as to where the future of psychiatry lay. Freud himself said that future psychology would probably be based on the "organic substructure" of the human body. The first half of the twentieth century certainly seemed to confirm this forecast, with Jacob Klaese and his prolonged sleep experiments in 1920, Sackels' insulin-induced coma in 1933, and the coming of electroconvulsive therapy (ECT) introduced by Ugo Cerletti in 1938. Some of these techniques have proved of value, though the much-publicized prefrontal lobotomy of Egar Moriz, also first attempted in 1938, is now rarely used.

Since World War II, and since the accidental discovery of the effect of LSD on the brain in 1943, great attention has been paid to the isolation of the active chemicals found in certain plants long used by ancient cultures to produce hallucinatory effects. Nearest to LSD is mescaline, the active ingredient of the peyote cactus, and also important is bufotenin, from the sacred mushroom of the Aztecs. From this it would seem apparent that, as Freud forecast, the future of psychiatry lies not so much in the analysis of mental states and behavior, but rather in the field of physiology and biochemistry.

XIV

The Herbalists

ONE OF THE delights of exploring any great city is the discovery of the old and picturesque cheek by jowl with the new and garish. London, perhaps more than any other capital city, is full of such surprises, and it therefore does not seem odd that just off the aggressively modern Kings Road in Chelsea we should find a three-hundred-year-old walled garden devoted entirely to the cultivation of herbs. This is the Chelsea Physic Garden, once the private garden of the fashionable London physician, Sir Hans Sloane (1660–1753), and medical adviser to Queen Anne. This is one of the few remaining examples of the herbal gardens once found all over Europe when it was commonly supposed that the Lord had provided the appropriate plant to cure every known remedy.

This belief was an ancient one. Nearly five thousand years earlier, about 3000 B.C., the Chinese Emperor Fu Hsi is thought to have been the first to investigate the science of agriculture and legend tells that so interested was he in the action of plants For this reason he was known as "the Heavenly Husbandman," and legends tells that so interested was he in the action of plants that he replaced part of his stomach wall with a section of glass the better to examine the workings of his digestive system.

Though Chinese medicine later evolved to incorporate such techniques as acupuncture, moxibustion, and pulse diagnosis, interest in herbs and medicinal plants did not cease, and by the

sixteenth century the Chinese physician Li-Shih Chen had devoted most of his life to writing a fifty-two-volume encyclopedia
of materia medica which listed nearly two thousand different
plants with appropriate prescriptions for virtually every known
illness.

In India, too, hundreds of plants were used medicinally,
some of which, after being neglected for centuries, are now receiving the attention of modern pharmacologists. Such a plant is
the climbing shrub, Rauwolfia, first mentioned by the Indian
physician Charaka in the second century A.D. He recommended
its use in intestinal diseases, fever, and snakebite, and it was also
popular as a specific for restlessness and insomnia. The plant was
rediscovered by the German doctor and explorer Leonhard Rau-
wolf (1540–1596) and given the name Rauwolfia, in his honor,
by a later researcher, the French monk and botanist Charles
Plumier, in 1703. In the late 1930s the properties of Rauwolfia
began to be investigated in laboratories in Europe and America,
and in 1949 its value as a hypotensive in the reduction of blood
pressure was finally confirmed. This was found to be due to the
presence in the plant of the alkaloid reserpine, one of about
twenty alkaloids finally isolated from Rauwolfia. The continued
use of reserpine, notably in the treatment of mental illness since
1954, demonstrates yet again that medical progress should not be
wholly concerned with the invention of new drugs, but should
include the thorough investigation of ancient remedies.

A further example is the four-thousand-year-old use of oil
from a Chinese fir tree in the treatment of bronchitis and asthma.
Not until 1878 did researchers discover that the beneficial powers of this particular plant product were due to the presence
of ephedrine, now accepted as a standard drug in the treatment
of pulmonary disorders.

As we have seen, medical history demonstrates, time and time
again, that while doctors were available to treat both the rich
and the very poor, the ordinary man had little access to them in
most countries. Ordinary people had recourse to herbs and plants,
whose properties were recognized for thousands of years, and
every cottager had part of his garden devoted to the growing of
such herbs to provide an appropriate remedy for every illness.
Faith in many of these plants was founded on experience and, as

has since been discovered, on the presence of some active ingredient unknown to the user. The diuretic action of the dandelion (known in French to this day as *pis-en-lit*) was founded on observation and experience, though its fame for imparting great physical strength does not rest on such a firm foundation. In many instances faith in a plant was based merely on the doctrine of signatures. In this way the little eyebright flower, looking like an eye, was used in an infusion to improve the sight, though there was nothing in the flower itself which could possibly be beneficial. In the same way the adder's-tongue fern was cultivated for the use in snakebite and in soreness of the tongue, while as far back as the first century A.D., the physician Dioscorides recommended the pink juice of the alkanet plant to cure pink sores on the skin. Similarly the use of pennyroyal tea to drive away fever and rheumatism was urged by Pliny the Elder in A.D. 70, with the added bonus that it also kept fleas away.

While the ordinary men and women of Europe made use of this vast armamentarium of herbs and plants available on the continent, exotic spices from the Orient were also being used medicinally and handled by specialist importers. From the twelfth century, huge trading caravans from China were traveling laboriously along the famous "silk roads" of the East, bringing drugs and spices to Bukhara, in Central Asia, from where they eventually reached Europe via the Black Sea. It was through a desire to obtain easier access to the Orient, and so facilitate the importation of spices, that the first tentative efforts were made by the Spaniards in the fifteenth century, and by the Dutch and British in the sixteenth and seventeenth centuries, to find a new route eastward by circumnavigating the globe. The result was the discovery of the New World.

Once travelers began returning to Europe from the Americas, many new plants were seen which had hitherto not been available in Europe, and many properties were attributed to them that did not exist in fact. Cocoa was first highly prized as a medicine, so was sarsaparilla and tobacco was considered a useful drug though highly intoxicating. Oddest of all, early in the seventeenth century the humble potato was in great demand as an aphrodisiac.

This period also saw the publication of books in several

countries attempting to classify and catalog the plants currently used in medicine.

The earliest printed English herbal was that of Richard Banckes (1525), followed the next year by *The Great Herball* of Peter Treveris. Neither of these was an original product; they were rough translations of earlier works on plants dating from the tenth century, or from French and German texts. German herbals in particular were known for the beauty of their illustrations, the most famous being that of Leonhard Fuchs printed in 1542. Fuchs, a noted Flemish botanist, gave his name to the fuchsia plant. Later, in 1551, the British botanist William Turner used many of Fuchs's illustrations in his own *Newe Herball,* which he dedicated to Queen Elizabeth I.

By far the best-known and best-loved of all the English herbalists was John Gerard (1545–1612). Born at Nantwich, in Cheshire, he was for many years head gardener to the powerful Cecil family during the reign of Elizabeth. He traveled widely, studying plants and their actions, and became a member of the Barber-Surgeons Company in 1595. In his London garden he had cultivated over a thousand different medicinal plants, many of them sent to him by friends and acquaintances he had met while traveling abroad.

In 1597 he wrote and published his herbal, a work which became immediately popular not so much for its accuracy (which was wanting in many respects) but for the enormous range of its contents, for its charm, and for its humor. Its inaccuracies were later corrected, and the whole work revised, by Thomas Johnson in 1636, but it is as *Gerard's Herbal* that the work is known and loved throughout the civilized world. A recognized authority on herbals and their authors, Miss E. S. Rohde, has described *Gerard's Herbal* thus in her *The Old English Herbal* (1922):

> His Herbal gripped the imagination of the English garden-loving world, and now, after a lapse of three-hundred years, it still retains its hold on us. There are English-speaking people the world over who may know nothing of any other, but at least by name they knew Gerard's Herbal. . . . One reads his critics with a respect due to their superior learning, and then returns to Gerard's Herbal

with the comfortable sensation of slipping away from a boring sermon into the pleasant spaciousness of an old-fashioned fairytale. For the majority of us are not scientific, nor do we care very much about being instructed. What we like is to read about daffodils and violets and gilliflowers and rosemary and thyme and all the other delicious old-fashioned English flowers. And when we can read about them in the matchless Elizabethan English we ask nothing more.

Gerard's book is dedicated to his former employer, William Cecil, Lord Burghley, then lord high treasurer to the queen. In his introduction he says:

> To the large and singular furniture of this Noble Island I have added from forreine places all the varietie of herbes and floures that I might any waye obtaine, I have laboured with the soile to make it fit for plants, and with the plants, that they may delight in the soile so that they may live and prosper under our clymat as in their native and proper countrie; what my success hath beene I leave to the report of they that have seene your Lordship's garden, and the little plotte under myne owne care and husbandry.

Gerard lists some two hundred plants, giving for each its description, normal place of cultivation, alternative names, and finally the "vertues" found in it. Conscious of the mass of folklore surrounding the use of herbs, he is scathing about some of the more outlandish fables which persist, such as those connected with the mandrake plant.

> There hath beene many ridiculous tales brought up of this plant, whether of olde wives or some runnagates Surgeon or Physick-mongers I know not, (a title bad enough for them) but sure some one or more that sought to make themselves famous were the first brochers of that errour I speake of. That it is never or very seldom to be found growing naturally, but under a gallows, where the matter that hath fallen from the dead body hath given it the shape of a man, and the matter of a woman the substance of the female plant; with many other such doltish dreames. They fable further and affirme: That he who would take up a plant thereof must tie a dog thereunto to pull it up, which will give great shreeke at the digging up; otherwise if a man should do it, he should surely die in short space after. Beside many fables of loving matters, too full of scurrilitie to set forth in print, which I

forebeare to speak of. All of which dreames and olde wives tales you shall henceforth cast out of your books and memory; knowing this, that they are all and everie part of them false and most untrue; for I myself and my servants also have digged up, planted and replanted very many, and yet never could perceive shape of man or woman. . . .

On the other hand some of Gerard's own claims seem a little farfetched, as, for example, his description of the "vertues" of onions. According to him, "Mixed with Salt, Rue or Honey, and so applied, they are good against the bite of a mad Dog," and again, "The juice of Onions anointed upon a pild or Bald head in the sun, bringeth the haire again very speedily."
"Clownes Wound-wort or All-Heale" (*Stachys palustris*) he describes how an ointment which will cure almost every kind of wound can be made from the juice of the plant. Evidently he once met a countryman who had sustained a wound from his scythe but who insisted on treating himself. Says Gerard: "I saw the wound and offered to heale the same for charity; which he refused, saying that I could not heale it as well as himselfe: a clownish answer I confesse, without any thankes for my goodwill: whereupon I have named the plant Clownes Wound-wort, as aforesaid."

On the topic of the recently discovered tobacco plant, Gerard is very voluble, and the description of its "vertues" runs to nearly four pages. Taken internally, he maintains, the juice is good for migraine, for toothache and for "dropsie." It also could be used as an antidote to all poisons. It can be smoked: "the dry leaves are used to be taken in a pipe, set on fire and suckt into the stomache, and thrust forth againe the nosthrils, against paines in the head, rheumes or aches in any part of the body."

Finally, says Gerard, "Many notable medicines are made hereof against the old and inveterat cough, against asthmaticall or pectorall griefes, all of which if I should set down at large, would require a peculiare volume."

As an Elizabethan gentleman of some substance, Gerard was fond of good living and did not stint himself. But as a doctor he warns against the excessive use of alcohol in a footnote to his description of the cultivation of the grapevine:

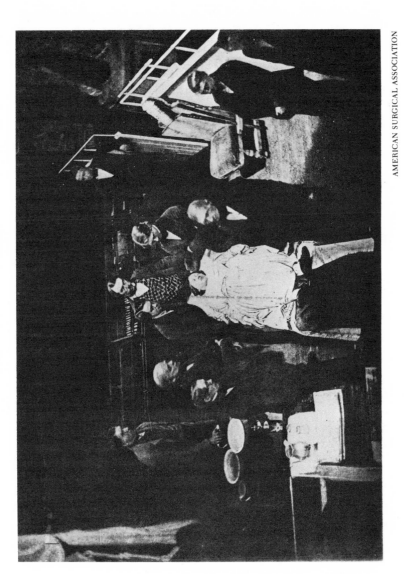

One of the first operations using ether as an anesthetic. Photographed at the Massachusetts General Hospital in 1846.

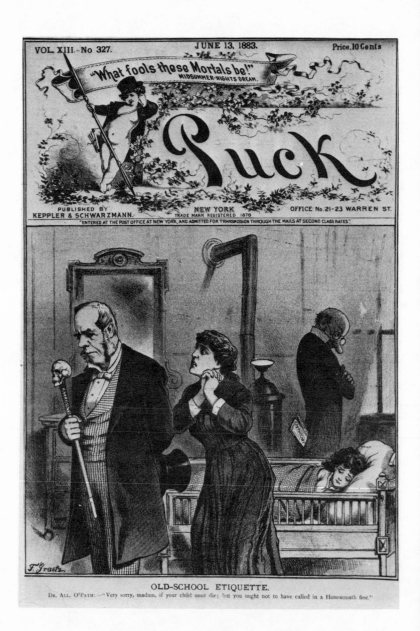

Cover of the magazine, *Puck*, of June 13, 1883. It was captioned:
Dr. All O'Path:—"Very sorry, madam, if your child must die; but
you ought not to have called in a Homeopath first."

Almighty God for the comfort of mankinde ordained Wine;
but decreed withall, That it should be moderately taken, for so
it is wholsome and comfortable: but when measure is turned into
excesse, it becommeth unwholsome, and a poyson most venemous.
Besides, how little credence is to be given to the drunkard is
evident; for though they may be mighty men, yet it maketh them
monsters, and worse than brute beasts. Finally in a word to con-
clude; this excessive drinking of Wine dishonoreth Noblemen,
beggereth the poore, and more have been destroied by surfeiting
therewith, than by the sword.

John Gerard, as much for his style as for the information he
supplies, remains a vivid and much-loved figure, but he was by
no means the only herbalist of his day.

Thirteen years after Johnson had published his 1636 edition
of *Gerard's Herbal*, a book on similar lines was produced by that
flamboyant and colorful figure, Nicholas Culpeper. He, too, was
a physician in the City of London and was also well-known as an
astrologer. He was a graduate of the University of Cambridge,
was highly proficient in Latin and Greek, and thought by many
of his contemporaries to be too clever by half. At any rate the
publication of his medical herbal, titled *A Physickal Directory*,
in 1649 immediately created trouble for the author. He was accused of pirating the Latin *Pharmacopeia* of the Royal College
of Physicians and translating into English without permission.
Not only that, but Culpeper introduced his own comments and
criticisms regarding some of the college's most cherished beliefs,
and held them up to ridicule. But far worse than any of these,
Culpeper revived the earlier theory that astrology had a powerful influence on the healing powers of plants, and they should be
collected and gathered only when the stars were favorable. This
was a theory propounded by John Bankes, a noted herbalist of
his day, a century before, and which had never been accepted
by the College of Physicians.

The college was enraged and acted quickly against Culpeper.
Unfortunately their method of attack was on personal lines
rather than on scientific ones, and they accused Culpeper of
being a drunkard and a lecher (which he probably was), rather
than combat his criticisms with arguments of their own. The
result of this was a vast amount of publicity for Culpeper and his

book, ensuring that it would be read and studied for the next three hundred years.

Another famous botanist and traveler was John Tradescant, head gardener to Charles I. His 'physick garden" in Lambeth, South London, was famous for the subtropical plants he had brought back from Africa and which he succeeded in growing there. Yet another favorite of the king, John Parkinson, wrote his own herbal in 1629 and was appointed botanist royal to the king.

Since those times many new herbals have been written, but those later than the seventeenth century have added little to the total sum of knowledge regarding healing plants. Only when new herbs and plants were still arriving from overseas was it possible to experiment and make fresh discoveries, and such research was actively encouraged by various learned societies. Indeed, it still went on until the end of the eighteenth century when the Royal Society of Arts in England encouraged investigation into the then little-known rhubarb plant from Russia and China. (Just why the Royal Society of Arts should have been so interested in rhubarb, rather than the botanists or physicians, remains a mystery.) At all events, after some rhubarb seeds had been successfully smuggled out of Russia to England in the diplomatic bag and distributed to members, the society, in 1770, promised a gold medal to any person raising more than one hundred plants in one season.

The prize was won several years in succession by Thomas Jones, a pharmacist of London who, on his ground at Enfield, eventually succeeded in rearing a forest of five thousand rhubarb plants. Fortunately for him, what Gerard would have called "the vertues" of rhubarb were by then well-known, and highly valued by doctors, enabling Jones to sell his entire crop each year to half a dozen of the main hospitals in London and to the value of five hundred thousand dollars.

The eighteenth century was the era of heroic doses and polypharmacy—the inclusion in one prescription of up to twenty different ingredients to make sure that some worked. It was inevitable that there would be a move back to simpler forms of medication and more natural methods of treatment, and in 1747 this was sparked off by the publication of John Wesley's book, *Primitive Physick*.

Wesley, in his role as a religious leader, moved constantly among ordinary people who were much influenced by him. In his introduction to *Primitive Physick: Or an Easy and Natural Method of Curing most Diseases*, he leaves the reader in no doubt at all as to his views on doctors and druggists. He says:

> And against the greater part of these medicines there is a further Objection: They consist of too many ingredients. This Common Method of compounding and decompounding medicines can never be reconciled with Common Sense. Experience shows that One Thing will cure most disorders at least as twenty put together. Then why do you add the other nineteen? Only to swell the apothecary's bill: Nay, possibly on purpose to prolong the distemper, that the Doctor and he may divide the Spoils.

These are, perhaps, somewhat uncharitable thoughts for a man of God, but Wesley was not a complicated individual, and for him things were either black or white. Many of his remedies were sound and taken straight from the pages of great herbalists. Wise, too, was his injunction that all writing should be done standing up at a tall desk. Other recommendations were less usual, such as his "cure" for tuberculosis, consisting of digging a hole in the turf, lying down, and breathing into the hole for fifteen minutes.

Yet another of his cures for this disease, though sounding equally farfetched, is now known to have a scientific basis. This was for sufferers from tuberculosis to "suck the milk of a healthy woman daily." Modern research now indicates that Wesley was on the right lines here, for human milk has now been shown to be a powerful inhibitor of the tubercle bacillus, against which cows' milk is powerless. Less scientific, but still perhaps of some value, is Wesley's "cure" for madness, which consists of making the sufferer wear a hat full of snow for three successive days!

Today, though polypharmacy is now a thing of the past, there is a renewed movement back to "primitive" medicine as a reaction against modern drugs and their many side effects. Herbalists have been with us continuously for many centuries, but in the twentieth century tend to be looked down upon by the

medical profession who prefer the complex but controlled drugs
of the pharmaceutical laboratory. Certainly it is true that a patient with a heart condition should be prescribed a precise and
accurate dose of digitalis, rather than swallow the distilled juice
of a pound of foxgloves, but the older remedies can still play a
part and should not be overlooked.

In Eastern countries there is a much closer relationship between herbal medicine and modern drugs than exists in the West,
and the pages of a periodical such as *Japanese Medical News*
will carry advertisement for herbal cough mixtures and cardiac
stimulants side by side with those for the most modern and sophisticated drugs.

The giant Takeda Chemical Company of Japan, for example,
has not only one of the most modern pharmaceutical research
laboratories to be found, but at Kyoto has the world's largest
herb garden. Here plants can be grown under ideal conditions,
and their properties and ingredients tested and assayed in the
laboratories. Plants like garlic, ginseng, and cinchona are still
being studied in order to grow them in such a manner that the
active principal of the plant remains at its maximum, at its pur-
est, and at its most stable.

Traditional herbs can still produce surprises, as the Takeda
chemists well know, and in addition the herb garden can provide
a valuable testing ground in the evolution of better and more
efficient weed killers and pesticides.

Western pharmaceutical companies could still take a leaf out
of the Japanese herb book in this respect, and benefit by it.

XV

The Doctor in the Twentieth Century

So RAPID HAVE been the changes in medicine this century, and so numerous the new drugs and treatments available to the patient and practitioner, that it is difficult to realize that the nineteenth century is still within the lifetime of an octogenarian.

Yet only a century ago, in many countries, the standards of medicine and medical teaching were abysmally low when compared with the situation today. This certainly applied to America.

In 1875, though several medical schools existed, the level of teaching was low and the standards required for qualifying were minimal. Baltimore, as an example, could boast five medical schools, but in the majority of them a medical qualification could be obtained after only two years' study and with the student never having seen a sick patient. Yet it was Baltimore that saw the greatest step taken in the improvement of medical teaching when the Quaker philanthropist, Johns Hopkins (1795–1873), bequeathed a large sum in his will for founding the medical school that today bears his name.

Later in the century the Johns Hopkins was to include those great figures of medical teaching known as "the four saints"— William Osler (1849–1919) from Canada, William Henry Welch (1850–1934) from Connecticut, William Stewart Halsted (1852–1922), the New York surgeon, and Howard Kelly (1858–1943), the Irish-American gynecologist. Under these men the standard of medical teaching improved tremendously at Hopkins, so much so that Osler was constrained to remark to Welch on one occasion: "We were lucky to get in here as professors; we would never have been accepted as students!"

Osler, a man of extraordinary and diverse talents, and not only a pathologist but a clinician, teacher, sanitarian, and expert bibliophile, made what was probably the greatest contribution to medical training at the time by insisting that fourth-year students should be in close contact with patients, and have real clinical experience before qualifying, instead of the theory and book learning that had gone before.

Meanwhile, in Europe, medical research was beginning to move away from the nineteenth century and enter a new phase. An early example was the evolution of the X ray.

In 1895 experiments were being made by a German doctor named Wilhelm Roentgen (1845–1923) on rays being produced by a gas-filled tube through which electricity was being passed (the Crookes tube). His experiments resulted in the discovery of a new kind of ray which he called 'X rays' because their exact nature was unknown. These rays, unlike light rays, could not be reflected by any substance nor could they be deviated by a prism. In addition, unlike the cathode rays of the Crookes tube, they could not be deflected by a magnet.

After announcing the discovery of his new rays in a lecture at Würzburg in 1896, Roentgen was besieged by the press, who took up with great excitement, and even greater inaccuracy, the fascinating story of rays which could pass through human flesh and reveal bone structures and fractures. So garbled were the press versions all over the world of the "invisible light" that revealed all, that writers wrote in indignation of the "revolting indecency" of an invention that made privacy impossible in the future. Underwear manufacturers tried to cash in on the new invention by advertising "X-ray proof" briefs and singlets, and in America, an Assemblyman named Deed attempted to launch a bill to "ban the use of X-ray opera-glasses in theaters."

The invention was of inestimable value to medicine, and with the use of bismuth, and later barium, X-ray photographs could be taken not only of bone structures but of the workings of the digestive system leading to the early diagnosis of gastric ulcers and other conditions. For this discovery Roentgen was awarded the Nobel Prize for physics in 1901.

Unfortunately it was not realized for some years that long exposure to X rays could precipitate cancer of the skin, and many early workers were martyrs to research. Later it was discovered that X rays could also be used as a therapeutic agent in the treatment of cancer, as well as a diagnostic technique, and today deep X ray therapy is a recognized part of the treatment of malignant disease.

Another weapon in the treatment of cancer was evolved by the Polish-French doctor, Marie Curie (1867–1934), and her husband Pierre Curie (1859–1906), working with radium in Paris. Further research was undertaken by the Curie's daughter, Irène Joliot-Curie (1897–1956), and her husband Frederic Joliot (1900–1958) when they observed in 1934 that aluminum bombarded with alpha rays produced artificial radioactivity.

Alongside research of this kind geared to the cure of known diseases, much work was continuing in the field of preventive medicine. In the late nineteenth century the French scientist, Claude Bernard (1813–1878) had studied the function of what he termed "internal secretions" which were later to be identified and classified as hormones. In the realm of nutritional research valuable contributions were made in London by Sir Frederick Gowland Hopkins (1861–1947) who discovered that health could not be maintained merely by ensuring a supply of synthetic calories and carbohydrates, but that the body required certain "food factors." These were later to be known as vitamins.

The early years of the twentieth century were marked by a great deal of research into the metabolism of the human body, and few discoveries were of such importance as that of the identification of insulin by Sir Frederick Banting (1891–1941) and his assistant Charles Best (1899–) in the treatment of diabetes. After several years of experimentation, they successfully proved the existence and action of the hormone insulin, working in the Toronto laboratories of Professor John James Macleod (1876–1935). In 1923 the Nobel Prize for physiology and medicine was awarded to Banting and Macleod, a decision which precipitated much argument and dissension, as Macleod had only lent his laboratories and had worked on insulin with Banting only after its discovery had been announced. Charles Best, who was not included in the award, had worked with Banting from the beginning. In any event, Banting decided to share his award with Best, and it is to these two men that the discovery of insulin is normally credited. The Nobel Prize Committee defended its action (or lack of it) by insisting that "technical reasons" prevented them awarding the prize to Best. It seems that nobody had remembered to nominate him!

The dawn of the twentieth century also demonstrated an increasing concern in many countries with public health schemes. Germany had been a pioneer in national health insurance, and in 1883 had introduced the compulsory insurance of industrial workers against sickness. The medical profession was deeply divided over this measure, and at first a feature of the scheme was the long and acrimonious disputes between the profession and the government over such matters as the remuneration of doctors and the freedom of the patient to chose his own practitioner. But agreement was eventually reached, and by 1911 insurance in Germany included not only sickness but also accidents and an old-age pension.

This was basically the system adopted in Britain in 1911 by Lloyd George, the fiery Welsh politician, and the scheme was later extended by another Welshman, Aneurin Bevan, in his National Health Scheme of 1948.

The development of medicine in Europe and America changed gear dramatically soon after the end of World War II. Prior to this event doctors on both sides of the Atlantic had been content to write prescriptions for the old and accepted remedies whose efficacy had been proved time and time again. Pharmacists filled prescriptions for iron salts for anemia, valerian and bromide for nervous conditions, bismuth and gentian for digestive troubles, and a whole range of vegetable compounds of doubtful value for colds and bronchitis. In the 1930s doctors still wrote "real" prescriptions, selecting ingredients and working out dosage and frequency. Suddenly things began to change.

In 1936 the second International Congress for Microbiology

was held in London, at which a doctor from St. Mary's Hospital, Paddington, read a paper on the bacteriostatic action of a certain mold called *Penicillium*. The doctor was Alexander Fleming (1881–1955), who had first noted the properties of the mold in 1928 and published a paper on it. But neither then, nor at the congress in 1936, was much importance given to the discovery, and it was not until the outbreak of World War II in 1939 that a new impetus was given to research in the battle against bacteria. At this point two researchers at the University of Oxford, Howard Florey (1898–1968) and Ernest B. Chain (1906–) went back to Fleming's discovery of 1928 and undertook further research which resulted in the isolation of the active principle of the mold, named by them as penicillin.

Wartime Britain was not conducive to scientific research of this kind, and the work was transferred to the United States where the first successful reports of the use of penicillin appeared in 1941. Fleming, Florey, and Chain were awarded the Nobel Prize for Medicine in 1945, and since that time a vast range of associated products, known generally as antibiotics, has come into use in the treatment of infections.

One of the most important of these after penicillin was streptomycin, evolved by the American scientist Selman Waksman (1888–), researching at Rutgers University in 1948. In 1952 he, too, was awarded the Nobel Prize.

One of the reasons why Fleming's discovery was not afforded much attention at the 1936 conference in London was because the proceedings were largely dominated by the new and exciting discovery of the sulfonamides.

Work on this group of chemicals had begun in 1904 when the German bacteriologist, Paul Ehrlich (1854–1915), had investigated the close affinity existing between some microorganisms and certain aniline dyes. Research was continued by his pupil Gerhard Domagk (1895–1964) and the publication of his findings in 1935 heralded the arrival of the sulfonamides, which were to be such an important force in the treatment of tuberculosis.

Since the end of World War II the accent has been on chemotherapy, or the action of synthetic chemicals on disease (of which Paul Ehrlich is considered to be the founder), with pharmaceutical firms in Europe, Asia, and America all producing a vast armamentarium of chemical compounds to alleviate, if not cure, virtually every known disease. International drug companies compete with each other in the sale of their own "ethical" products (products largely obtainable only with a prescription and advertised only to the medical profession), many of which duplicate each other. In some instances more than thirty forms of the same drug, in the same dosage, are available under different trade names for the treatment of the same condition. This creates problems for the general practitioner in his ultimate choice of product. In the end, he is inclined to use the product of the firm whose name he knows best, which is usually the product whose originator has expended the most money on publicity and promotion.

This vast and extensive range of modern drugs available, together with new techniques such as vaccination for whooping cough and measles, new drugs for hypertension, and improved diagnostic techniques, are of the utmost importance to the doctor in his daily practice. Other developments, like organ transplants, neurosurgery, psychosomatic treatment, endocrinology and research into genetics are of passing interest. He knows they are available, but the average practitioner is dealing with far less dramatic conditions in his normal work.

He is concerned with coughs and colds, with indigestion and constipation, with "nerves" and depression and at all times with birth and death. He gets disillusioned, he gets tired, he gets worn out (the death rate from cardiac failure is significantly higher among doctors than in other professions), but at all times he must be able to hold out hope, if not for a permanent cure, at least for some symptomatic relief.

Though the concept of the family doctor is tending to become less definite, in most countries its continued existence depends on the way medicine operates and on what sort of national health service is in existence. There is much variation in this.

Britain's National Health Service, existing in its present form since 1948, is simplicity itself as far as the patient is concerned. From the pay of every employed and self-employed person in Britain the sum of about five dollars is deducted weekly to cover sickness, unemployment, and social security. Once that is done, the person who falls ill has nothing further to worry about financially. Medical attention by a doctor is free, the services of consultants and specialists are automatic and free (if the doctor thinks they are neccessary), and hospitalization and operations are free. For the patient the system is a good one and compares favorably with other national health schemes in operation.

In France, for example, the patient must himself pay the doctor, the druggist, the ambulance, and the hospital, and then reclaim the expense incurred by filling countless forms and waiting for anything up to six months. Even then he does not recover from the state the total amount expended, but a proportion varying between 65 percent and 95 percent according to the urgency and nature of his illness. To pay the balance the Frenchman has recourse to private insurance schemes based normally on his trade or profession and geared to his earnings.

In Britain every doctor under contract to the National Health Scheme is paid the annual sum of eight dollars for every patient registered with him, whether he attends him or not. Critics of the scheme outside Britain maintain that the system is unfair to the healthy patient, who is made to subsidize the sick one. This is not really so. The deduction of five dollars from his weekly wage is a standard amount and does not vary according to how often other people need medical attention. Furthermore, those who are fortunate enough to remain healthy do not begrudge the amount deducted, for they know that even if part of that sum (for it also covers unemployment benefits and social security) represents medical attention that they do not require at the time, it needs only one comparatively serious illness and a bout of hospitalization to show them a handsome profit.

What the patient in Britain complains about today is the increasing difficulty of access to his doctor and his reluctance to call on the patient at his home. During the last ten years the British family doctor has slowly been engulfed by work, with more and more consultations and a corresponding cut in the amount of time he can allow any one patient. As several consultations at the office can be made in the time it takes to visit one patient, doctors are actively discouraging patients from expecting to be visited, and virtually compelling them to attend the office.

The British public, reared in the old tradition of the family doctor coming to the house, is at present resisting this tendency, but it is fighting a losing battle. Parents still expect the doctor to attend their sick children, and are understandably annoyed when they are told to bring the children to the office. For this reason the relationship between British general practitioners and their patients has been deteriorating, a situation not improved by the evolution of the medical center, staffed by up to six doctors, and the possibility of the patient being seen by a different doctor each time he attends.

Unlike the system obtaining in America and in some European countries, the British general practitioner does not follow his patient into the hospital. There is, too often, an almost complete shut-off once the patient is hospitalized, and many doctors complain of the difficulty of obtaining information about their patients, and in particular the time that elapses between the sending home of the patient and the receipt of instructions regarding follow-up treatment.

A valid criticism of the British National Health Insurance scheme is that it encourages hypochondriacs and those with only trivial complaints to rush to the doctor, something they would never do if they had to pay for treatment, even if they recovered it later. The early hope that a free health service would result in improved health nationally has not been justified. People are not less ill (though the pattern of illness has changed) but they go to the doctor more. This fact, coupled with the availability of free medication and treatment to visiting foreigners, is one of the reasons why British general practitioners are extended to their limit.

While nobody wants to change the basic concept of a free health service for all, changes are coming in the organization of the scheme. Most important is the evolution of the medical care team, consisting of doctors, nurses, and social workers, which will deal with 90 percent of all cases, sending only 10 percent on to the consultant who works mainly through the hospital. This will mean a fundamental difference in the training of doctors and will (it is hoped) create a breed of practitioner who is, in fact, a "specialist" family doctor with a training as rigorous as that at present required by a surgeon.

In most countries the tendency to specialize is increasing. If this continues, and if specialization comes to include the former general practitioner, the concept of the old family doctor will have gone for good. The famous bedside manner so valued in the past will be needed no more. Doctors will no longer attend patients in their homes (as has already happened in some countries) and the specialist will be king.

Whether this is a good thing or not is a matter of debate. One of the troubles about overspecialization, where people are trained to perform only specific jobs, is that eventually there will be nobody left to perform the common tasks.

In America in particular this has resulted in a scarcity of doctors in the more remote and rural parts of the country. In West Virginia, as an example, Doddridge County, an area covering 320 square miles but with a population of only 6500, has had no doctor for two years. Even before that time few doctors stayed very long, the last one leaving and retreating to university life on the grounds that the work he was required to do was well below that for which he had been trained. This pattern is being repeated throughout the United States, and Doddridge County is only one of 145 counties throughout America which have no doctor.

Changes are on the way and there are at present (1976) twenty bills concerned with federal health programs before Congress. Plans include a funding system and payment to doctors by means of which they would be spread more evenly where they are wanted. At present New York State has one doctor to every 500 population, whereas in South Dakota it is one to 1500. It is hoped that the scheme will iron out such anomalies.

There is another scheme (which has already started) by which medical students, usually in their final two years, can obtain government grants covering living expenses and tuition, in return for which they agree to go to areas where there are no doctors.

If changes of this kind come about, places like Doddridge County, where there is no doctor and where many folk have a three-hour journey to a hospital, will finally get the medical care to which it is entitled. There is no point in governments priding themselves on the quality of life, liberty, and happiness without the realization that none of these are possible without good health—and that means adequate medical attention for all.

But what sort of medical attention is going to be available? Patients are changing, not only in their attitude toward doctors, but in the kind of attention they expect to receive from them. There is, for example, much evidence that people today have a far lower threshold of tolerance to ill-health than formerly. "What the patient wants today," says an experienced practitioner, "is the promise of the elixir of life. But in addition he wants papal dispensation to go on doing all the things we have warned him not to do for his health's sake."

The resounding failures of the antismoking propaganda in Britain and in America and the government antialcohol campaign in France are good examples of this.

The practitioner of today is increasingly expected to advise on the emotional problems of his patients. While the trained psychiatrist may be a specialist in schizophrenia and other well-defined disorders, the average practitioner is becoming more and more a specialist in unhappiness. He is finding that what presents itself as a physical disturbance can often be diagnosed as stemming from an emotional one. This is one aspect of doctoring in which few practitioners are adequately trained as yet. As the medical teaching revolution gets under way, it is to be hoped that this situation will be rectified. As was recently remarked: "The family doctor must deal with the emotional stress as devotedly as with the physical damage. His fundamental job is to try and love the human being."

In the final analysis, most doctors succeed in doing this. It is their love for their fellowmen that underpins the whole relationship between doctor and patient, which makes it vitally important that this relationship should have the means and opportunity to develop and mature.

At the beginning of this book we quoted the Hippocratic Oath that governed medical conduct in ancient times. In 1948 in

Geneva the World Medical Association evolved a modern version of this oath. We cannot do better than end by quoting it:

THE GENEVA DECLARATION

At the time of being admitted a Member of the Medical
    Profession:

*I solemnly pledge myself to consecrate my life to the service
    of humanity;*

*I will give my teachers the respect and gratitude which is
    their due;*

*I will practice my profession with conscience and with
    dignity;*

The health of my patient will be my first consideration;

I will respect the secrets which are confided in me;

*I will maintain by all the means in my power, the honor and
    the noble traditions of the medical profession;*

My colleagues will be my brothers;

*I will not permit considerations of religion, nationality or
    race, party politics or social standing to intervene between
    my duty and my patient;*

*I will maintain the utmost respect for human life from the
    time of conception; even under threat I will not use my
    medical knowledge contrary to the laws of humanity;*

I make these promises solemnly, freely and upon my honour.

Selected Bibliography

Bailey, Thomas A. *The American Pageant*. Boston: D. C. Heath, 1966.

Barber, Geoffrey. *Country Doctor*. Ipswich, England: Boydell Press, 1968.

Bashford, A. *The Harley Street Calendar*. London: Constable, 1929.

Baumber, E. *In Search of the Magic Bullet*. London: Thames & Hudson, 1965.

Block, Marc. *The Royal Touch*. London: Routledge & Kegan Paul, 1971.

Bondi, E., ed. *The Story of Medicine*. London: Marshall Cavendish, 1968.

Brain, Lord. *Doctors Past and Present*. New York: Pitman Medical, 1964.

Brander, Michael. *The Georgian Gentlemen*. Lexington, Mass.: Saxon House, 1973.

Camp, John. *Magic, Myth & Medicine*. New York: Taplinger Publishing, 1974.

Davidson, M. H. A. *The Evolution of Anesthesia,* Altrincham, Cheshire, England: John Sherratt, 1965.

Deux, G. *The Black Death*. London: Hamish Hamilton, 1969.

Guthrie, D. *The History of Medicine*. London: Nelson, 1945.

Haggard, A. W. *The Doctor in History*. New Haven, Conn.: Yale University Press, 1934.

Haggard, Howard W. *Devils, Drugs & Doctors*. New York: Harper & Row, 1975.

Jameson, Eric. *The Natural History of Quackery*. London: Michael Joseph, 1961.

Lane, K. *The Longest Art*. London: Allen & Unwin, 1969.

Levey, J de B. *Illustrated Herbal Book*. London: Faber & Faber, 1974.

Lloyd, M. *A Hundred Years of Medicine*. London: Duckworth, 1936.

Macalpine, Ida, and Hunter, Richard A. *George III and the Mad Business*. London: Allen Lane, 1969.

Maple, Eric. *Magic, Medicine and Quackery*. London: Robert Hale, 1968.

Marti-Ibanez, F., ed. *The Pageant of Medicine*. London: Gollancz, 1960.

Matthews, G. *The History of Pharmacy in Britain*. Edinburgh: Livingstone, 1962.

Mayo, Charles W. *Mayo—The Story of My Family*. New York: Doubleday, 1968.

Mitchell, L. C., ed. *The Purefoy Letters*. London: Sidgwick & Jackson, 1973.

Munthe, Axel. *The Story of San Michele*. London: John Murray, 1929.

Office of Health Economics. *The Health Care Dilemma*. London, 1975.

Palos, Stephan. *Chinese Art of Healing*. New York: McGraw-Hill, 1971.

Pickering, George. *The Creative Malady*. London: Allen & Unwin, 1974.

Pollack & Underwood. *The Healers*. London: Nelson, 1968.

Pound, R. *Harley Street*. London: Michael Joseph, 1967.

Robertson, G. G. *Gorbals Doctor*. London: Jarrolds, 1970.

Rosenberg, Charles. *The Cholera Years*. Chicago: University of Chicago Press, 1962.

Segrist, E. *The Great Doctors*. Translated by E. Paul. New York: Dover Publications, 1971.

Singer, Charles, and Underwood, Ashworth E. *A Short History of Medicine*. New York: Oxford University Press, 1962.

Sitwell, Edith. *English Eccentrics*. London: Dobson Books, 1958.

Talbot, C. H. *Medicine in Medieval England*. London: Oldbourne Book Co., 1967.

Turner, E. S. *Taking the Cure*. London: Michael Joseph, 1967.

Venzmer, G. *5000 Years of Medicine*. Translated by M. Koenig. London: Macdonald, 1972.

Wilson, C., and Pitman, P. *Encyclopedia of Murder*. London: Arthur Barker, 1961.

Woodward, Marcus. *Gerard's Herbal*, 1936 ed. New York: Minerva Press, 1971.

Wykes, A. *Eccentric Doctors*. Oxford, England: Mowbrays, 1975.